IN STITCHES

The Highs and Lows of Life
as an A&E Doctor

Dr Nick Edwards

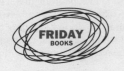

FRIDAY
BOOKS

The Friday Project
An imprint of HarperCollinsPublishers
77–85 Fulham Palace Road, Hammersmith, London W6 8JB

www.thefridayproject.co.uk
www.harpercollins.co.uk

This edition published by The Friday Project 2011

1

First published in Great Britain by The Friday Project in 2007

A catalogue record for this book is available from the British Library

ISBN 978-1-905548-70-5

*In Stitches is not authorised or endorsed by the NHS and opinions expressed
within this book do not reflect those of the NHS. All situations and characters
contained within the book are amalgamations of different scenarios at different
hospitals and names and timing have been changed to protect anonymity. The
author would like it to be known that he is writing under a pseudonym.*

Set in Times New Roman 11/14.5 by Wordsense Ltd, Edinburgh

Printed and bound in Great Britain by Clays Ltd, St Ives plc

Mixed Sources
Product group from well-managed
forests and other controlled sources
www.fsc.org Cert no. SW-COC-1806
© 1996 Forest Stewardship Council

FSC is a non-profit international organisation established to promote the
responsible management of the world's forests. Products carrying the FSC
label are independently certified to assure consumers that they come
from forests that are managed to meet the social, economic and
ecological needs of present and future generations.

Find out more about HarperCollins and the environment at
www.harpercollins.co.uk/green

IN STITCHES

The Highs and Lows of Life
as an A&E Doctor

03809366

To Mrs Edwards: Thank you so much for everything; from making me laugh, to bringing into the world our two kids and helping me back down to earth by rolling your eyes when I talk with an overinflated ego.

Disclaimer: this book is an attempt to take a humorous look at what it is like to work in a British Accident and Emergency Department. Much of it is tongue in cheek, so do not use it as a guide on how to manage illnesses. Call your GP or, if you can't be bothered to wait for their receptionist to answer the phone, call an ambulance and come on down to your local A&E department for 3 hours and 59 minutes of fun.

Preface

It is 4 years since I wrote *In Stitches*, the highs and lows of life as an A&E doctor. During that time so much has changed, to me, to my outlook and to the way A&E departments and the wider NHS are run. One thing that hasn't changed is the enjoyment I get from the challenge of treating the variety of patients that come to A&E. Often after a hard day at work, I will complain that it was the same shit just another day. But stepping back, it is the variety of shit, the way it is dumped out and the different ways we flush it away that makes this job so interesting.

When I was asked by my publisher if I wanted to update the book, the first thing I did was re-read the first edition. Initially I wanted to change most of it. I was a moany git, who pontificated on micro-management and was a bit self-righteous. But it was written as a blog-style diary and so changing what I wrote then would distort the original book. So when you read the book please bear this in mind.

At the end of the second edition is an 'epilogue': what I have been up to for the last 4 years, a few of my thoughts and my favourite stories and vignettes from working in A&E during that time. I hope you enjoy both the original book and the additions for the second edition. Thank you for reading.

Introduction

It was a fairly standard Saturday at work; generally busy and stressful but interrupted by episodes of upset, excitement and amusement. However, being honest, I quite enjoyed myself. I found pleasure in successfully treating someone's heart failure and liked being able to mend a patient's dislocated shoulder. I was amused by a drunk and injured tough-looking biker-type who had got into a fight over a game of chess. And I had a quite fascinating conversation with a man in his late 80s (who came in after a car accident), who insisted on telling me about his current sex life difficulties. Overall, if you have got to work, then working in A&E (Accident and Emergency) is one of the most interesting jobs I could think of and I am glad that it is the job I do.

Admittedly, I got mildly frustrated by the sheer number of patients who were revelling in the British culture of getting as pissed as possible, starting a fight and then coming in to A&E. And yes, I got a little weary of seeing a number of patients who had not read the big red (and quite explicit) sign as they walked in, and who had neither an accident nor an emergency and should have seen an out-of-hours GP (if one had been more readily available). However, overall, I saw a lot of patients who genuinely needed our services and whom we could help, which is the bit of my job that I love.

There was one patient that I took an instant liking to. She was in her mid-80s and had such a fast wit and spark to her personality that she felt like a breath of fresh air as I was treating her. She touched my emotional heartstrings because she reminded me of my Great Aunt.

She came in after having collapsed at home with abdominal pain, vomiting and diarrhoea. We were busy and she had had to wait 2 hours to see me. I quickly made the diagnosis of a possible gastro-enteritis (stomach bug), gave her some fluids, took some blood, organised an X-ray and arranged for admission. I wanted to wait for the results, spend more time with her and manage her care accordingly, but in a flash she was whisked away to a care of the elderly ward for me never to see her again. An hour after she arrived on the ward (and before she was seen by the ward doctors), she suddenly deteriorated and her blood pressure fell. This wasn't noticed as quickly as it might have been had she stayed in A&E as the ward nurses were so rushed off their feet (two trained nurses having to look after 24 demanding patients).

She had been rushed out of A&E to get her to a ward so that she wouldn't break the government's 4-hour target (and because the A&E department has not got the resources to continue safely caring for patients for longer than a few hours in addition to seeing all the new ones constantly coming through the doors). I also had to pass responsibility over to the other doctors before her blood tests were back and before a definitive diagnosis was made. I later learned that she had been anaemic, which had put stress on her heart, and that she then ended up on the high-dependency ward, needing a blood transfusion.

For a while it was touch and go as to whether she could be stabilised. I couldn't help wondering whether, if she had remained in A&E, under our care, all these problems could have been treated sooner and the complications avoided. However, this was not possible as, apparently, I had more pressing priorities. My next job was to go and see a bloke who had called an ambulance to get his ingrown toenail looked at and who had been waiting for 3 hours. He had, incidentally, had this problem for five weeks and wanted it (in his words) 'sorted out now, as I'm off to Ibiza tomorrow, mate'.

I felt really frustrated. It didn't need to be like this. Why does the 'system' have to impede me from caring for my sick patients and make me worry about figures and targets instead?

When you are surrounded by death and disease, aggressive and drunk patients, and nurses (male and female) trying constantly to flirt with you, it can make working in A&E an interesting and often stressful environment. However, it is the management problems and the effects of the NHS reforms, implemented without thinking about the possibilities of unintended consequences that really drive doctors and nurses mad. More importantly, they distort clinical priorities and can damage patient care. Surely this is not what the government intended? How have we drifted away from the original ideals of the NHS?

In July 1948, Nye Bevan presided over the creation of the NHS. It is a service that provides free care based on need and not ability to pay; to care for us from the cradle to the grave. It was the envy of the world and the greatest example of social policy this country has ever implemented. It is a wonderful institution that needs protecting and nurturing. Its desire to protect health and not profits means that its efficiency could outstrip that of any other health system in the world. The very thought of working for it filled me with pride.

By 1997, years of underfunding had left the NHS in a perilous state. Massive influxes of money from Blair and Brown poured in, which helped bring in some great improvements in service and much-needed reforms. This is especially true in A&E, where things have improved greatly from the days of patients spending days in corridors on trolleys waiting for a bed. The target brought in was a 4-hour rule stating that 98 per cent of people have to be seen and admitted or discharged within 4 hours. Initially, it was a necessary but blunt tool, which effectively brought about urgently needed change. However, its lack of subtlety and implementation without resort to common sense is now impeding care and distorting priorities.

Despite the enormous sums of money that have been spent, for the NHS as a whole the overall benefits have been underwhelming. In the last few years, the government has managed to demoralise a significant number of hospital workers despite these huge increases in resources. To try and get 'better value for money' targets have been implemented and reforms made that threaten the structure, efficiency and ethos of the NHS, driving it away from cooperation and caring towards incoherence and profit making. For those of us who believe in the idea of collectivism enshrined in the NHS, it is a worrying time. It is an especially worrying time if you live near a hospital that is under threat of closure or losing its A&E in the name of 'reforms'.

These worries about what is happening to the NHS (and in particular A&E) combined with the general demands of the job, can sometimes make me feel a bit stressed. Many people cope with this by drinking; however, I usually have to stop after a pint, as I start to feel sick and get a rash. Instead I started ranting to my friends and moaning to my wife: she started to threaten divorce and my friends seemed to invite me out less and less. So, in an attempt to save my sanity and marriage, I turned to writing down my frustrations with the job. A cathartic form of literary therapy.

That is, in part, what this book is about. It is a collection of stories written to try and explain what working in A&E is really like. It is not just about the frustrations – far from it. I have also tried to provide a small indication of the buzz I get from work and the amusement and banter that can be found there, including the dark humour that is used to cope with the stress of the job. I have tried to describe the joy I get from observing the eccentricities of the human condition and the fascinating little ironies life throws upon us. I have, in addition, tried to cover more serious aspects of the problems facing today's NHS and A&E departments in particular. All the stories are typical of ones retold in staff coffee-rooms up and down the country. They are based on events that have happened to me, or colleagues, working in various hospitals throughout the last six years. However, details have been changed and the stories described are often an amalgam of many similar incidents rather than one specific case. If you think you recognise a clinical situation or problem, it is probably because it is repeated daily in all A&E departments.

This book is certainly not a whistle-blowing exercise, as the situations described are universal problems and not specific to one hospital. I certainly feel that the departments I have worked in are good and the consultants have been supportive. The way they manage to provide top-quality clinical care despite the management concerns occurring in the background, provide me with appropriate role models. Neither is this book a blog as such (although the idea started out as a blog) – there is no real-time order to the various passages. There is no underlying story and neither are the stories arranged into any theme. It is just a random selection of events and experiences as an A&E doctor.

I hope you enjoy reading it – both the amusing and sarcastic bits and the ones where I am being serious. I hope to inform you what really goes on in your local A&E and what the people working there are going through, so that if you happen to need our services, you will understand when things don't work as smoothly as perhaps they should. The views and ideas in the book are my own and are not endorsed by any political organisation or pressure group. I am not a politician or a manager, but I do work on the 'coal face' of the NHS and can see its problems.

I don't think the NHS is having its best year ever. I think all the recent reforms and targets and private sector involvement are really making things go a bit 'tits up'. I want to share with you some of my concerns and how they affect my working life, as well as showing you the real highs and lows of life as an A&E doctor. Thank you for reading.

Dr Nick Edwards, July 2007

P.S. For those of you who want a quick summary of what life is like working in A&E, without having to read the book, then here goes. It is a bit like what you see on TV programmes such as ER, *but with less sex and more paper work. I, unfortunately, do not look like George Clooney either – more like Charlie out of* Casualty. *I have also never asked for a 'chem 20 stat' and the medical students are not usually as beautiful or as helpful as the ones depicted in* ER.

A sign the world has gone mad?

What was happening to my patients today? They seemed to be getting lost when I sent them for X-ray. I'd given the same directions as normal, there had been no secret muggers hiding in the hospital corridors and, as far as I know, no problems with space–time dimensions in our particular corner of the universe.

I went to X-ray to investigate. I found it quickly because I knew the way. However, I looked for the signs for X-ray and they were gone. The nice, old-fashioned and slightly worn signs had gone; they had been replaced by a sign saying 'Department of Diagnostic Imaging'. What the hell? *I* know what it means, but only just, and only because I have been inundated by politically correct 'shit-speak' for a number of years. What a pointless waste of money; to satisfy some manager, they replaced a perfectly good sign with one that means bugger all to 90 per cent of people. Why don't they change the toilet sign to 'Department of Faecal and Urinary Excrement' or the cafe to 'Calorific Enhancement Area'? Who makes these decisions? Who is employed to do such pointless stuff? Why? Why?? Why???

I needed a caffeinated beverage in a disposable single-use container – management-speak for shit NHS/Happy Shopper instant coffee. I went to sit in the 'Relaxation, Rest and Reflection Room', previously known as the staff room.

There, the nurses were moaning that one of their colleagues had called in sick tonight and to save money their shift would not be covered by an agency nurse. In A&E, staff shortages can seriously undermine the safety of patient care.

I am sure this genius plan was decided by some personnel manager who I doubt has ever seen a patient, cannula or trolley, and is therefore obviously an expert at making nursing planning decisions. So we have a hospital that can fund unnecessary new signs, but not replace nurses when they are off sick. So, tonight who is going to go looking for the patients when they get lost en route to the Department of Diagnostic Imaging?

Management madness

If politicians tell you that by instilling the ethos of the private sector we can improve the efficiency of the NHS and improve patient care, then let me tell you that is rubbish. What is needed is good old-fashioned common sense and cooperation. Unfortunately, this is difficult to put on a balance sheet.

Let me give you an example that really upset me. An old man who had Alzheimer's and was in a nursing home tripped and fell and banged his head. He was on his way to the toilet, but had forgotten that he normally needed a frame and a nurse to help him. He sustained a laceration to his forehead. He needed five stitches, and then to go home. He arrived at 11 p.m.

It was a very quiet night. I was asked to see him straight away as the nurse in charge knew that we could discharge him back very quickly. Fifteen minutes later he was ready for discharge and the ambulance crew that had brought him in were still having a chat and coffee with us all. The charge nurse asked if they would take him back and they didn't mind at all. They called the coordinator at the control centre (someone who has never worked on an ambulance). He told them that they couldn't take the patient back to his nursing home, as our hospital (to save money) had changed the terms of contract with the ambulance trust and no non-essential transfers were to be done after 11 p.m. The ambulance man protested and explained that there were three ambulances in the locality, all with their feet up. He said he didn't mind doing it as it was for the old man's benefit. Control responded with a statement about breaking contractual obligations, setting a precedent and influencing future contract negotiations.

Further protests ensued. The man was not safe to get a taxi on his own but was still well enough to go back to his nursing home. There was a willing crew who were free at the time and I couldn't see the problem. I tried to intervene and told control about how the man was confused and distressed about coming into hospital. I explained that staying in hospital until 9 a.m. the next morning would make him worse. However, I was told that the 3 per cent funding shift resource allocation caused by the contract change had meant that they could no longer do goodwill gestures such as I had requested.

It was ridiculous. For no good reason beyond disjointed management decisions – made introspectively, without thinking about the consequence for the whole NHS – this man had to stay in an A&E ward for 10 hours. He became very upset and distressed. A&E later became much busier and our nurses didn't have time to take him to the toilet and so he soiled himself. He screamed all night because he was confused and disorientated in this strange place and the patients in the bed next to him slept very poorly. I was then asked to prescribe sedatives for the patients in the A&E ward, and for him!

I just don't understand what is happening in management; I don't think that management understands what is happening on the A&E 'shop floor'. I found out from one of the senior A&E nurses that the contract decision was changed to save a very small amount of money. Managers would have slapped themselves on their backs for their 'efficiency' savings to the transport budget, but not realised that it would not have saved the hospital, or the NHS as a whole, a single penny (the patient still needed to go back in the morning!).

I was annoyed with our managers, but why did the ambulance control man act in the way he did? A few years ago, the crews would have taken these patients back if they were quiet – contract or no contract – for the good for the patient. I suppose nowadays people are instructed to do stuff only if it is for the good of the targets and common sense has flown out of the window.

I got very stressed and angry about this. After a while the junior doctor working with me asked why I was so irate. I explained that, apart from an irate personality disorder and the fact that ranting is my form of therapy, I was genuinely upset. Apart from my lovely family and useless football team, the things I care most about are my patients' care and the state of the NHS. It upsets me that crappy management decisions done in the name of 'efficiency' bugger up both.

P.S. If there are any politicians/managers wanting to see the actual effect of NHS policies (both good and bad) on patient care, please ask your local A&E department if you can spend a night working alongside the doctors and nurses. You will learn more about the problems in that one night, than you ever will from looking at a balance sheet or 'throughput' data that A&E departments send their hospital managers.

P.P.S. If you think I will only ever talk about how awful things are, please be assured that some things have improved dramatically over the last few years, it is just that I want them to continue improving and not get worse again. Also, when there are no problems, I do not get angry and so do not feel the need to write. So, if you think everything I say is biased, then, yes, you are right. But biased for the right reason: to try and get things changed for the better... and to help with my stress relief.

Treating your own family

It is a well-known fact that you should not be a doctor for your family. This is true. I certainly found out how true last night...

It was the quietest night we had had for a long time. A&E was empty when my wife's grandpa arrived. He is in his 90s, demented, and spending the last few years of his life in a confused state in a nursing home. The staff at his nursing home had called an ambulance as he was more short of breath than usual.

I got the other doctor to see him and told them all his problems. I explained that on his previous admission, the consultant had declared him 'Not for Resus' (i.e. if his heart were to stop, then it would not be appropriate to try to restart it with cardiopulmonary resuscitation – CPR). This was the right thing because his quality of life was so poor. In all honesty, I just hoped for his sake that he would pass away peacefully in his sleep. I had a chat with him and then, when he fell asleep, I left to get a drink. It was very quiet in A&E and he was the only one left in the department.

I was dozing in the coffee room, when the alarm call came through the intercom. 'Cardiac arrest, Resus'. I ran there past where Grandpa was meant to be. He wasn't there. For Christ's sake! Why had they moved him into the Resus room, and why were they doing something futile and cruel? I was livid.

I ran into the Resus room. Everything went into slow motion. There was a nurse jumping up and down on an elderly man's chest and the doctor ventilating his lungs. I was furious. 'Let him die in a dignified way and not with broken ribs,' I thought.

'STOP. STOP. BLOODY HELL, STOP', I screamed.

'It's not your grandpa, Nick. He has gone for an X-ray. This bloke just collapsed in reception about twenty seconds ago.'

'CONTINUE, CONTINUE', I screamed back. 'BLOODY HELL, CONTINUE.'

Ridiculously embarrassed, I managed to regain my composure and lead a successful cardiac resuscitation. We got back a pulse and called the anaesthetists to take over his breathing. He went to ICU (the intensive care unit) and three weeks later was discharged to lead a normal life. Thank God everyone ignored my advice to stop.

Meanwhile, my wife's grandpa was sent back to his home the next day and is still in the same sorry way.

ℓ Dealing with threatening patients

I get scared sometimes at work. I work in a rather tough town – even the muggers go round in pairs. Consequently, we get some rather tough patients. Give them some alcohol and they become a little hostile. Add the stress of waiting 3 hours and 59 minutes and they become aggressive. The fact that they are often in A&E because they lost a fight sometimes results in them looking for revenge – and A&E staff are often the target.

I am a not a 'weed' but I am not sure that I could handle myself if I ever got into a proper fight. With a lack of any training in self-defence, and an A&E security guard that my Nan could 'have', you sometimes feel a little vulnerable. I have never been assaulted but I know a number of colleagues who have. The BBC programme *Panorama* investigated this violence and reported that a NHS worker gets attacked every 7 minutes. However, much of the 'violence' results from the confusion caused by medical problems. I have been bitten by a lady in her 80s who was short of oxygen. It wasn't her fault – it was probably mine – I should have been more careful. When she was better she was the most beautifully placid person in the world. These are not the type of 'violent' patients that upset me. It is the aggressive, bullying types who know all their rights but have no sense of respect that irk me and make my job scary at times.

Last night I was at the desk, writing my notes, when a drunk and aggressive man came up to me and was forcibly complaining that I was delaying his treatment because I was being anti-Moldovan. (Maybe I need to go on a cultural awareness course, because I didn't even realise he was Moldovan or, more to the point, where in fact Moldovia is.) All I knew was that he was a man who did not need to be seen before the bloke who need 15 sutures for a bottling injury and who was bleeding profusely.

The patient became very aggressive and angry. As he started to walk menacing towards me, I started to apologise profusely (as well as sweat profusely). Experience has taught me that this often stops aggressive people in their tracks as they are frequently expecting a fight back. Worth a try, I thought…

'I am very sorry sir, but we are very busy tonight. We see people in order of priority and not time order, I am afraid.'

He kept shouting insults and making demands. He was not happy with his wait. Eventually, it was obvious my tactic was not working. I just wanted to ask him to leave in a firm way, but I was too scared of him. Luckily, I could see that there were two policemen in the waiting room, who had 'smelt' trouble and had started to walk towards me. I breathed a sigh of relief and suddenly found lots of bravado.

'I am very sorry', I said, before adding 'for having to take your insults. I have been working ridiculously hard all night and don't deserve your language or behaviour.'

My temper now started to rise. 'If you dare speak to anyone like this again you will not be treated. Now sit down and be quiet and wait your turn. If you have a problem with this, then leave.'

I pointed to the door and felt like a brave warrior who had just defended his tribe of A&E doctors and nurses, but I knew that I was a warrior of the type that only stands up for himself in the presence of a policeman. In reality, I am still a scared wimp who is polite to rude and threatening patients purely because I am afraid of breaking my General Medical Council code of ethics of treating people in a non-judgmental way... and because I don't want my head kicked in.

On one occasion when someone would not stop complaining and became verbally threatening, my colleague took them to the door of the resuscitation room to show them what we were doing and why his wait was so long. The complainer commented that it wasn't his problem and later wrote a complaint letter about the psychological upset he had been subjected to. Unfortunately, my colleague has not felt compelled to be brave enough to do this again and now just ends up apologising behind gritted teeth.

It is very difficult dealing with violence in hospitals. What do you do with an injured patient who needs your care but is threatening? It is easy if they have assaulted someone as you can call the police. But bullying and threatening behaviour is difficult to deal with. Personally, I think it is time that in addition to patients having more and more rights, NHS workers had more rights and protection too – they certainly need it. Unfortunately, we have become too politically correct. The modern NHS thinks of patients as customers and we are encouraged to believe that 'the customer is always right' but sometimes that is just not the case.

℞ No notes

The ambulance pulled up and the paramedic came out. 'Nick, we need to take him to Resus. His pulse is only 30.' It seemed a reasonable request so I went off to Resus to see him.

The patient was 80, lived alone and had no close relatives. He had dementia and received care four times a day. The carer had called the 'out of hours' GP because his catheter was blocked, he couldn't pass urine and his stomach was starting to ache. The GP told them to come to A&E as the out-of-hours service was too busy. A much better course of action would have been for them to go and 'unblock' the catheter, but that is a moan for another day.

I examined him and, apart from having a blocked catheter, the main problem was his pulse of 30 (normal is about 60). His ECG showed 'complete heart block', a condition that makes the heart beat very slowly. His blood pressure was normal, so it wasn't an immediate life-threatening event, but heart block can be very serious, particularly if it is a new condition.

I asked the patient about it. He didn't really understand what I was talking about. The carer didn't know. I phoned the out-of-hours GP, but they can't access regular GP notes outside working hours. The carer didn't know anything about his heart condition, and there were no relatives available to ask. I asked our receptionists to get his old notes urgently as I needed to know what was going on. Would he need to go to the cardiac unit urgently or could he go home?

The A&E receptionist said that she couldn't get hold of the notes. They were in a secretary's office awaiting 'typing' and no-one could get hold of them. I moved on up the food chain and called the hospital 'Site Manager', the most senior person present in the hospital in the evening.

'I need them urgently', I pleaded.

'Unfortunately, we can't,' I was informed.

'It is life threatening. Please can we get them?'

'Computer says no' (OK, she didn't actually say that, but it was something to that effect).

I had to practise safe medicine, so I referred him to the medical doctors to be monitored on the cardiac care unit (CCU). I explained that I thought it was a chronic problem, but that I wasn't prepared to take the risk. They agreed and he went to the CCU.

In the morning, when the cardiologists were debating what to do, the GP was called and the hospital notes obtained. It was soon found that he had had this condition for five years. He had been referred for a pacemaker, but had refused one as the condition had never bothered him. The GP also explained that when the patient had been 'with it' he had always said that he never wanted to go for a hospital for a pacemaker. This pretty much swung the treatment plan into discharging him back home.

However, this visit put him at risk of hospital-acquired infection, and took up the last bed on the CCU, which might have prevented someone who would have genuinely benefited from coming to CCU from being there. And why? Because we couldn't get hold of his old notes outside office hours. It is so frustrating to work in a system like this – what a waste of money. This happens time after time after time – unnecessary admissions occur, expensive tests are repeated and patients are not being cared for properly – all because of poor accessibility of patient records.

The government sees that this is happening and that is why it is currently spending zillions and zillions of pounds on a new computer system. Unfortunately, this system is taking ages to be implemented. Until it is, couldn't we do something like, say, getting GPs to give every patient/or their carer a summary of their notes to carry around with them? Currently, even if I can get hospital paper notes, I can't get access to GP records of patients' latest drugs

Going back to the computer system they are implementing, I say thank you. It is about time too, but why is it taking so long and why the hell is it costing so much? I know it is complicated, but all I want is a system where a patient comes in with an NHS ID card, we swipe it and know what medications they are on, what they are allergic to, any past medical conditions and, perhaps, get a copy of an old ECG. And when they get a new condition or drug change, the doctor can change the 'care record' then and there.

We don't need some fancy thing with 'choose and book' and Internet blardy, blah, blah. We just need something that works and we need it now. If Tesco can know exactly what I have bought every week for the last few years and have brought that IT system in at a fraction of the cost of the NHS's one, can't we steal their IT manager? Or Sainsbury's Nectar card computer bod? Without easy access to patient records, we provide worse and more expensive care. Hurry up computer people, please.

Off duty?

Tonight I saw three bad knees and three sore throats, and had a discussion about the pros and cons of being referred for a hip replacement. I was asked about how to stop the symptoms of the menopause and what to do for dry vaginas. I was asked about how to stop babies crying and if I could listen to someone's heart and feel their pulse as they had been having palpitations… Yes, I was at my mum and dad's Boxing Day party.

Please, friends, just let me drink and talk about beer and football. It's my day off. I want to have a laugh and joke and not talk about your ailments.

An upsetting day

I had a real low day at work today. I saw two really upsetting cases that I am sure will stick in my mind for a long time. A 13-year-old girl was brought in by her dad. She was complaining of abdominal pain, had been missing school and waking up in the night crying out because of the pain. The dad had brought in his child during one of these episodes as he was at the end of his tether.

The child had variable symptoms and signs and none pointed to a specific organic pathology. I asked her if she was upset about anything – she denied this and got very annoyed. I asked the dad if I could talk to the girl in private just in case there was something she didn't want her dad to know; again, she denied any reason for stress. However, the dad came back into the cubicle and with a tear in his eye told me that his wife had died six months previously and that his daughter had not come to terms with it – she had barely shed a tear. It confirmed my belief that all her pains were being expressed via medical symptoms – this is called somatisation. The pain is real and is certainly not the same as malingering or factitious behaviour but is very hard to treat as it requires psychological rather than physical treatment. This poor girl had genuine abdominal pain that no medication could cure.

I am not sure if it was the right thing to do, but I did a battery of tests to prove that nothing was wrong. They all came back normal and I told her so and discharged her, then advised her dad to try and take her to her GP to arrange some grief counselling or something. I hope she is all right in the future – I'll never know. This is something that makes me a little jealous of GPs – they get to see and shape what happens with their patients. I only get to see them in times of crisis and often never know if I've made a difference or not.

The next patient made me even more distressed. She was a lady in her 80s who was brought in by ambulance after becoming increasingly short of breath. She came in with her husband of 58 years. She had been very unwell the last five years since suffering a stroke and then having a series of mini-strokes causing a form of dementia (called multi-infarct dementia).

The husband had refused all previous plans to put her in a nursing home, as he had made a promise to her five years ago that he would look after her himself. She was immobile, incontinent and had severe dementia, but he had still kept to his word. Day after day he lovingly cleaned her, cooked for her and held her hand and talked to her. He was an angel in every sense of the word.

Before the ambulance arrived, we had got a call explaining that they thought she might have suffered a respiratory arrest (i.e. stopped breathing). As soon as she arrived, I could see how unwell she was. My SHO (junior doctor) gave oxygen and fluids and organised a chest X-ray, while I talked to the husband.

It soon became clear what the situation was. Taking over her breathing and sending her to ICU was not an appropriate thing to do. It would be more humane to let her die peacefully. I explained this to the husband. He broke down in tears and just said, 'Thank you. I can't cope any more and nor can she.'

I smiled and invited him in to be with her. She spent the last few hours of her life held tightly by her husband, listening to him telling her how much he loved her and recounting all the good times they had in the past.

It was a sad but beautiful sight that I felt privileged to witness. Emergency medicine is not just about the high drama of trying to save someone's life. Sometimes the most important skill in medicine is knowing when to let nature take its course and not interfere. It was sad to see, but also the right thing to have allowed to happen.

Having to cope with the upset that these type of situations create is something that can never really be taught at medical school.

Right and left problems

I felt like a prat today. This eight-year-old boy came in after falling on an outstretched right arm. It looked like it was probably broken. I gave him my usual preamble with boys to make him feel at ease.

'So what football team do you support?' I asked.

'Man City', he replied. 'Joey Barton is brilliant,' he added. I told him my little joke about our hospital policy being not to treat Man United supporters as a way to save money. He laughed but I am not sure if his dad realised I was trying to be funny.

'Blimin' good idea that is. Bunch of pansies the lot of them.'

'Oh dear', I thought, and went back to examine the boy, then wrote an X-ray form. I wrote 'X-ray R wrist please'. I always try and be polite on my forms – it usually helps to oil the cogs of the working day.

He came back with his X-ray and to my surprise there was no fracture. I reassured him and his dad, and sent them on their way, with the advice he was to come back if it continued to hurt.

Seven hours later he was back – this time with his mum – and still in pain. As he was a returning patient, he had to be reviewed by a middle-grade doctor (like myself) or consultant. Luckily (for me and my blushes) it was after 6 p.m. and I was the most senior doctor around. I examined him again, and explained that muscle injuries can be just as painful as broken bones.

His mum then asked, 'Do you have a policy of only X-raying

the wrong hand if they support City, or does it not matter and you X-ray everybody's wrong hand?'

I was flabbergasted. I protested. Surely her son was making things up. I went and got the X-ray form to prove that I had written R on it. I had written R, but the radiographer had read L as, to be fair my R looked like a L. I looked at the X-ray – yes there was an obvious 'Left' written on it. What a dick I had been. I apologised to the mum profusely. A new X-ray form was written with 'Right' written instead of R and it duly came back with a small undisplaced fracture needing a plaster of Paris cast. Luckily, no harm was done.

I apologised, held my hand up and admitted my error. I told the mother that I was never going to write R and L again, but spend the extra second finishing off the word. She seemed to accept my apologies. She also wanted to clarify that her nephew would be able to come to hospital if he ever got ill. He is a Man United supporter. 'Oh dear', I thought, as I went on to explain myself for a second time.

A note to all readers. The Man United comment was meant as a sarcastic joke. All NHS hospitals will see supporters of any football club. Don't worry… well, unless you support Chelsea – then you are on your own.

℞ What a waste of talent

I am writing this passage with an almighty hangover. What a
night. We had a lot of celebrating/commiserating to do. Three
of my close colleagues are quitting work as A&E doctors. One
is retraining to be a GP, another is moving to Australia and my
third colleague is retraining to be a management consultant
– she doesn't want to give up medicine, but she has kids at
school and a mortgage to pay and is worried that she is going
to be unemployed in August, because of the uncertainty of the
new recruiting system. All are fed up with the lifestyle and the
way they are treated.

However, it is not just A&E where hospital doctors are
feeling fed up and angry. Hospital doctors, both junior and
senior, throughout the country are becoming more and more
disillusioned and are leaving in droves. These decisions have
been entirely justifiable for the individuals concerned, but for
the country as a whole it has been an enormous waste of talent
and money. This is happening at a time when more and more
money is being pumped into the NHS. How can this be? There
are a number of reasons, but ultimately it is because hospital
doctors are feeling undervalued and are being blamed for the
NHS's ills; they are fed up with poor working conditions,
ungrateful management and feeling unable to direct the
reforms occurring in the NHS. Tragically, there has been a
new way of recruiting junior doctors, which is impeding some
of our best-qualified and most experienced junior doctors
from getting jobs and thus forcing them to leave the NHS. The
problems for hospital doctors are exacerbated when they see

that even when they do qualify there are apparently going to be too many consultants and not enough jobs to go round. Will they finish all their post-graduate training to end up working only as subconsultants?

Junior doctors are feeling especially angry. It is true that there is no longer the ridiculous culture of 48-hour shifts. However, there are still unpleasant lifestyles associated with working as a doctor. Once qualified, there are the chores of having to rotate round various hospitals every six months, the stress of post-graduate exams and the worries of having to apply very frequently for new jobs. They say one of the most stressful events in life is moving and/or starting new jobs (along with getting married and having children). Junior doctors do this every six months – not the kids and marriage bits. The government has tried to rectify this by implementing changes to doctors' training but has only managed to demoralise a whole cohort of doctors in training (see next rant).

Hospital juniors are also getting annoyed because of the way they feel they are being treated compared with their GP colleagues. The GP trainees have much more training built into their rota, they get more supervision and are not just thrown into the deep end when they start jobs, as is sometimes the case with hospital jobs. Then there is the question of pay. I do not begrudge GPs their money – that much (the average GP does not earn as much as the press says), but when I am doing an A&E shift and a GP is doing a locum out-of-hours shift round the corner he is often getting more than treble my pay. When you know that, you feel undervalued and underappreciated. However, by comparison, I have absolutely nothing to complain about compared with the nurses, receptionists, cleaners, etc.

Consultants are also becoming more fed up and some are reducing their commitment to the NHS as a result. There are numerous reasons for this but they include disillusionment about the NHS reforms, loss of continuity of junior staff and having to work to artificial targets as opposed to clinical need.

The NHS is its staff. We need a hospital staff with high morale instead of this disillusionment we are all experiencing. It is not about money – it is about having job security, feeling valued and having our time and skills used appropriately... The only good news is that with more people leaving I am getting to go to more and more after-work drinking sessions. My wife can't really ban me if they are for long-standing colleagues' leaving dos...

MMC – mangling medical careers

A few weeks ago doctors organised a march against what the government is doing to junior doctors' training. I have never seen so many placid, conservative, non-volatile people on a demonstration before. They were campaigning against a programme called MMC – Modernising Medical Careers (otherwise known by some as demoralizing/mangling/ mismanaging medical careers). It certainly has benefits in terms of organising doctors' training from when they finish their 'foundation jobs' (the first jobs they get after qualifying). In A&E it has the added benefit of ensuring that every junior A&E doctor works for a time in anaesthetics and intensive care – jobs that are often hard to come by but that can teach you vital skills.

However, its implementation is what is really pissing off a vast number of doctors, damaging morale and, in the future, may damage patient care. Again, the intention was sensible enough – streamline doctors' training and try and make job opportunities fairer – but the implementation is farcical. Instead of bringing it in gradually, there has been a most ridiculous attempt to transfer a cohort of doctors from the old scheme to the new one at the same time as implementing the new training scheme for the very junior doctors. As a result 30000 doctors are applying for 22000 jobs.

It is the way that they are being forced to apply which is outrageous. The 'system' consists of a computer-based questionnaire that assesses your ability to write politically correct crap in 150 words. Doctors with experience, exams, research and wisdom are losing out to others who have been on a course on how to fill out the application form.

The lucky ones who are offered interviews are faced by senior doctors who have not seen their CVs and who have had to mark 600 applicants' forms in a weekend – but only one question on the form – and so they cannot possibly get an idea of the candidates. The lucky ones get jobs, but often in different parts of the country from where they live and where their kids go to school. They only get told about their jobs at short notice, then have to scramble to find somewhere new to live and somewhere to send their kids to school.

I know of so many doctors whose current contract is finishing in August and then do not know what they will do. Individually, it is upsetting; these doctors, who have debts from medical school and haven't hit high earnings yet, are left with the threat of no job and no future in the NHS. Collectively, it is a disaster; it costs £250 000 to train a doctor – we are losing thousands of doctors and that is millions and millions of pounds that we as the tax payers have wasted.

Tragically, no-one seems bothered. There is a campaign group (http://www.remedyuk.net) and a few Internet blogs that have taken a big interest such as http://www.drgrumble. blogspot.com. However, the national media has not seemed that concerned about the plight of the country's junior doctors and the fact that many of them are leaving the NHS at our expense.

How did this happen? I think it is government arrogance. They thought they knew best. They ignored the advice of the British Medical Association, which was to 'slow down, take stock and do this sensibly'. They rushed it through and now, despite a last-minute review, we are faced with this disastrous outcome. They then had the audacity to blame the senior doctors (via the Royal Colleges) who were the very ones urging caution against this whole system.

I know the politicians have said that doctors need to live in the real world and not expect a job for life and should expect competition for popular jobs. That is completely fair and in the past it was totally wrong that some doctors were helped by an 'old boys' network'. However it is the utter lack of care that the system shows for its employees that is upsetting. No other group of workers would accept such a shambolic arrangement: where thousands of junior doctors have had their contracts expire in August and then have to apply for new jobs where they can't show their CVs, don't know where they will work or what their pay or conditions will be. Then if they are lucky and get a new job, they will only have a couple of weeks notice to uproot themselves and their families before they start their new jobs – remember, this is not just happening to people just out of medical school, but to doctors in their mid thirties who have up to eight years experience and who have roots and families which they need to consider as well. The only people smiling at this mess are the employment lawyers who could be in for a windfall. Oh, and the Australian health service, which is getting loads of very good, well-trained doctors at the British tax payers' expense. No wonder the application system called MTAS (Medical Training Application System) has been nicknamed Migrating To Australia Soon.

P.S. Since this was written a review group have looked at how to try and improve everything. They are hatching a last-minute plan to try and save the government's blushes, and thousands of junior doctors' livelihoods. I wish them luck – they'll need it.

Still off duty?

When I am not at work, I love Saturdays. In the mornings I play for a local football team and in the afternoons I go with my dad to watch my apparently professional football team play in a depressive mid-season battle. However, this is only when the wife allows and so is becoming a rarer treat. Saturdays are now usually DIY-based – or screaming at some random IKEA instructions-based – as I fondly think of it.

But this Saturday I was allowed to play. We were playing top of the league and for those of us excited by regional lower division non-league football, boy, this was a big game. It started well. My fitness training had worked and I had played a blinder. One–nil down at half time had only spurred us on and with 15 minutes to go I had just scored a screamer from 40 yards to bring us level. The crowd was singing and I was feeling fantastic. Five minutes later, the ball came back to me. A one–two followed and we beat the offside trap. My mate sprinted forward. Rushing towards goal he was tripped. A penalty was awarded, but he was in agony. I ran forward and realised that his shoulder was obviously dislocated.

He was screaming and it ended up being my job to take him off the field and drive him to hospital, bypassing the queues and getting a friend to pull his shoulder back into position. But I didn't want to be there. I didn't want to be subbed just because I am a doctor. I wanted to score the winning penalty and then go to the pub afterwards. But alas no. I am still on duty even when I am out playing football.

P.S. My wife has just read this and has reminded me that this book is based on reality not fantasy. I must confess I hadn't done any fitness training, I was playing shit and we were 3–0 down and playing third from bottom – we are bottom. There was no singing from the crowd, just a bark from a random stray dog. The goal I scored was an own goal, which hit my bum as I fell over after my contact lens fell out. Sorry for the misinformation. The bit about the IKEA furniture and shoulder were true though. What is also true is that we both got back in time to join everyone for drinks. One perk of my job is that my mate bought my drinks for me to say thanks.

I want muffins

It was 6 a.m. and the canteen was closed. I was feeling hungry, having been on shift for 10 hours already. I went to help myself to a couple of pieces of toast. Admittedly, yes, technically it is for patient use, but it is one of the small perks of the job that we can get some free toast and tea in the early morning. This morning, on the front of the cupboard door, there was a new sign warning us that taking bread was theft and could end in disciplinary action.

Come on, who writes such ridiculously rude notes? Why, when managers are trying to save money, do they do pathetic things like take away tea and coffee and bread, and not look at really serious issues? I bet they had muffins at the meeting where they decided on this money pinching measure. If they are going to take away our bread, then let us have their muffins.

Bloody trains

For some unknown reason, I am on an eco-drive. I have spent a fortune on energy efficiency lights, become keen on recycling and started to come to work by train. I feel like an eco-warrior (a middle class one who is scared of climbing trees let alone living in one with a bloke called 'Swampy', but still in my eyes an 'eco-warrior'). I feel good about myself. These feelings vanish, however, as I get off the 8.42 train…

When I walked off the platform, there was a group of inspectors standing round a lady who was carrying a ridiculous number of bags. At first I thought she was shouting down a mobile phone. Then I realised that wasn't the problem.

'WHY DON'T YOU GET RID OF YOUR KNIVES?' She screamed in the general direction of the ticket inspectors.

'I KNOW WHY YOU WANT ME DEAD. BUT I DIDN'T CAUSE THE TRAIN CRASH.'

I approached and was told to stand back as she was apparently dangerous. She was very unwell, but, no, she wasn't dangerous. I recognised her straight away. She was in her 40s and was a known regular at A&E. She had mild learning difficulties and psychotic paranoia and depression; a diagnosis of schizophrenia had been made in the past. She had a problem with alcohol (i.e. she drank more than her doctor) and her coping mechanism for whenever she got stressed was to self-harm. For years she had been in and out of psychiatric hospitals, and was now receiving 'care in the community'.

In the past, patients like this may have been institutionalised, but they now are more likely to be cared for at home by community psychiatric nurses. However, these services are often under-funded and patients can slip through the 'care' bit of the 'care in the community' programmes. Instead, their 'care' is often provided by homeless shelters, police stations and A&E departments. This lady was one of these patients. She didn't cooperate with any of the programmes they had tried to involve her with. She was getting sicker living in the community, but there was little anyone seemed to be able to do for her. As a result she had been to A&E 78 times in the last four years.

I approached the ticket inspector who seemed to be in charge.

'What's going on?' I asked.

'Stand back. She is dangerous,' he told me, then started shouting at her: 'Lie on the floor with your hands on your head'.

'Bloody hell, she is clearly unwell but she's not a terrorist suspect,' I thought. She started screaming in fright and was scratching and biting herself to the point of bleeding. I intervened and called the police. I explained to the 999 control that this lady needed sectioning under 136 powers (i.e. the police could take her to a place of safety). When I explained that I was a doctor and not someone who needed sectioning themselves, they sent round two burly looking officers.

They were absolutely brilliant. They calmed her down and put her in the car while I unfolded my new bike and cycled to work – I really was on an eco-drive.

On arrival I explained why I had been late and that I had brought some work with me. This didn't go down well. As 'punishment', my task was to go and see the patient that I had just arranged to come in with the help of the boys in blue. As I went in to see her, I nodded in appreciation of their work earlier and started to speak to the patient.

'Hello. My name is Nick. I am one of the doctors here. What happened today?'

I said it in my most reassuring of voices, but it hadn't seemed to calm her down or helped with her paranoia at all.

'You aren't a doctor. You're a ticket inspector. I DIDN'T CAUSE THE CRASH. NOW GET OUT.'

Later that day, she was readmitted to a psychiatry ward. I saw her two weeks later, after another episode of self harm. It is a situation that we see all too often. In our current world of political correctness and not offering institutionalised care, there seems little we can do. As always, when there is a crisis, A&E is the point of call, but we cannot offer the long-term solutions that they need.

GP receptionists

I was sitting at the desk when this quite rude 45-year-old man marched up and moaned about how long he had waited and demanded to know if we were fulfilling government targets. (The answer, I thought to myself, was that he had not waited long enough as he should have been put to the back of the queue for being so pompous.) However, as he had a tie on and an aristocratic voice, everyone seemed to be getting a bit worried and I was asked to go and see him next. He had been suffering from pain in the wrist for three weeks. He had been doing a lot of typing recently and was suffering from 'tenosynovitis' (inflammation of the tendons). The treatment is a splint and painkillers.

I was a bit fed up that he had come to A&E with a chronic problem, so I asked him if he had looked at the sign outside and which bit of an accident or emergency he had. (OK, I didn't ask him that; I wanted to, but he had a suit and tie on and a posh voice and I didn't want a complaint letter. In fact, I just advised him that in future he went to his GP for this type of problem.)

I was a bit shocked when he told me what had happened. He went to his local GP and saw the receptionist, who demanded to know what was the matter with him. He told her and then *she* advised him to go to A&E as it wasn't 'the sort of thing' GPs do, despite his protests that he didn't want to go to A&E. (Despite being a doctor, I also get intimidated by GP receptionists demanding to know loudly what is wrong with you so the whole of the waiting room can hear. I once responded, 'I have got a growth on my dick, genital herpes and want a sex change, how about you?' and now they seem to let me see my GP without a CIA-type interrogation. This man wasn't so fortunate. He failed the interrogation and ended up in A&E – without an accident or emergency.) I had no option but to phone the GP. I got through to the receptionist and the conversation went a bit like this.

'Hi, could I speak to the duty GP please?'

'I am afraid he is on home visits all day, and then in a meeting so you won't be able to speak to him till at least next Thursday,' she responded.

'Sorry, I forgot to say my name is Dr Edwards. A&E registrar.'

'Oh… he is next to me. Having a cup of tea. Sorry, I errrr… forgot,' she responded.

I picked up the phone ready for an argument. I had all my lines prepared. I had real 'inappropriate attendee' rage (a bit similar to road rage, but with fewer horns). I thought the best line I had prepared was 'And what medical school did your receptionist go to?' I was ready to go. Start off calm and then let the battle commence…

He was brilliant. He had obviously been on a 'verbal judo/how to calm down irritated twats course', because he was magnificent.

'I am very sorry, Dr Edwards – I will look into it and retrain my staff as necessary. If you have any further problems, put them in writing. I would be most happy to meet you and discuss this issue face to face, etc., etc.' I wanted a bloody argument not an apology. I wanted to be able to moan and rant, but I ended up singing the GP's diplomatic skills. Maybe the reason he is so good, though, is because he gets so many complaints about his receptionists…

Why I love going to work

A set of seven nights and on night six I at last felt that I had done some genuine good and I remembered why I love going to work. At 1.30 a.m. a lady in her 70s came in peri-arrest (about to die). She had a blood pressure of only 60/30 and was becoming unconscious. We took her into Resus and while the nurses put in a cannula and gave her oxygen and fluids, I examined her and spoke to her husband. It was obvious that she had perforated her bowel and that she was losing fluid into her abdominal cavity.

Within half an hour, we had given her 3 litres of fluid and she was starting to perk up. However, she needed definitive treatment – a laparotomy (a major operation which would remove the damaged part of bowel and clear out the faeces that had leaked into her abdomen). I called the surgeons and anaesthetists and within half an hour she was in theatre. Two hours later, the perforated part of the bowel was removed and she was in the ICU. I phoned up the next day and she is doing so much better. A very good outcome as all of the A&E team worked very well with the surgeons and anaesthetist. Thanks to all of us, everything went perfectly and we saved her life –

you would be surprised how rarely we actually get to say that. All in all, it was a very satisfying night.

♀ This is how it feels like the NHS has been ℞ run the last few years

Gordon Brown pours money in. The senior nurses on the shop floor sensibly think we need more A&E nurses and so more are appointed. Then interfering politicians are concerned that the new nurses may not be very efficient and they are not getting value for money, so the managers appoint a 'staff efficiency evaluator' and a 'patient pathway flow monitor'.

This 'staff efficiency evaluator' and the 'patient pathway flow monitor' (separate jobs, mind) also need supervision and secretarial support, so a senior supervisor is appointed and a personal assistant. More money comes in from Gordon and so, to satisfy the finance departments, quarterly figures need to be produced on how efficient the new staff are, and how many 'direct patient contact' episodes are occurring. A business manager is appointed to the staff efficiency evaluation team for this purpose. So that the local hospital journal knows about how wonderfully efficient the new nurses are and how patient contact episodes are exceeding expectations (i.e. they have been told to document whenever they say 'hello' to someone) a marketing manager is appointed to the staff efficiency team. In truth, their job is to write a small article every two months for the pointless glossy-paged magazine that the hospital wastes its money on.

New concerns about the new nurses are brought up. Are they helping patients make choices to deliver a patient-centred care pathway? A patient-centred care pathway manager is appointed to the staff efficiency team. The election is over and the trust realises it has overspent vast amounts of money and now Gordon is not so friendly.

A 'turn-around' team are appointed at great expense. But they are geniuses and worth every penny of their grand a day. They show the light that no senior nurse or consultant could ever have seen. The answer is lying before our eyes... the nurses are not efficient enough, are not performing enough patient contact episodes and have lost focus on patient-centred care. An efficiency report is needed.

The report is produced – indeed, it is the workers' fault. The answer is patient-centred streamlined efficiency. This actually means they make the nurses redundant... but, remember, we couldn't possibly lay off the staff efficiency team as we will need to report to the finance team on how good our 'staff reorganisation initiatives' have been. We can't sack the marketing manager from the staff efficiency team as we need to tell people about staff reorganisation with a positive spin. The remaining nurses still need guidance and so the patient-centred care supervising manager needs their job protected. The business manager not only keeps their job, but needs a pay rise for doing extra work – handing out redundancy notices to the nurses.

♌ And this is how I would like the NHS to be managed

The Prime Minister says here is some money. New A&E nurses are employed. A senior nurse is appointed to monitor their progress and education. Patient care is improved and everybody is happy. No interference occurs from politicians. There are no massive overspends so brakes do not need to be applied (obviously only after an election). So, in summary, we can keep our nurses and let them do the job they were trained to do in the way they see fit. Oh! How I dream.

How does a government that has put so much money into the NHS (and it has), given pay rises and improved many services, still manage at the same time to piss off just about everyone that works in the NHS. It is an amazing skill. What it has done wrong is interfere so very badly in the micro-management of the NHS, arrange ridiculous targets aimed at winning elections and not long-term improvement in patient care, and disengage clinicians from involvement in management. Then there is the problem of pointless involvement of the private sector making profit out of the NHS…

What also pisses me off is when the Tories have their 'NHYes' campaign and say that they are the saviours of the NHS. Remember, they very nearly completely buggered it up. Don't forget the perilous state they left it in 1997.

What it seems to me is that neither party can be trusted to run the NHS. The NHS needs policies designed to look after health now and in the long term. It should not be used as a political football with short-term plans introduced for when general elections are due. We need the politics taken out of the NHS. Make it a semi-autonomous organisation, where management input comes from frontline medical/nursing trained staff and not management accountants (I am not so sure what they actually do). It needs to be run along the lines of the BBC – with guaranteed funding and an independent management board. Whichever party promises that, then they will get my vote.

P.S. Just had to let all the anger out – I just read in the local paper that my hospital was about to make lots of nurses redundant and I got upset.

Ooops

Examining females is always difficult for a male doctor. I always take a nurse with me as a chaperone – it makes it easier for the patient and less stressful for me.

About a year ago, an attractive 21-year-old teaching assistant was rushed into the resuscitation department. She was having breathing problems and her heart was running very fast. I examined her and could hear a heart murmur. This was very unusual for a young patient. I asked her if she could take off her top so I could examine her in more detail.

I put my hand at the apex of the heart – to medical people it is the fifth intercostal space mid auxiliary point. In normal language, it means I put my hand under her left breast. I closed my eyes as I tried to feel for the rushing of blood caused by the murmur – knowing if you can feel the murmur helps to grade its severity. The medical term for a palpable murmur is a 'thrill'. It feels like a vibration within the chest. It was hard to feel and my hands must have been underneath her breasts for at least 20 seconds. She looked at me nervously, so I tried to reassure her. 'Don't worry – I am just feeling for a thrill… '

Shit! That came out wrong, very wrong! Stuttering, I tried to explain myself – but I don't think that I managed to dig myself out of the hole very well. I stabilised her medical problem and referred her to the medical doctors for investigation and an echocardiogram. I wrote down the name of my chaperone very carefully. A year later I haven't heard anything, so I think my faux pas has been excused.

Where have all the dentists gone?

If you needed a plumber urgently, would you call out an electrician because there was a lack of plumbers in the neighbourhood, just in case they could sort you out? No, it is madness. So then why, oh why, do patients with toothache go to A&E. GO TO A BLOODY DENTIST. I know very little about teeth. Very few doctors do. Don't come to me with teeth problems, go to a dentist.

I got so annoyed with a man this morning – luckily I didn't show it, as it turned out he was blameless. We were very busy and I felt he was wasting our time. Instead of letting a steam rush come upon me, I tried to have a chat with him (more to calm me down). I asked him why had he come here. The answer surprised me. It wasn't NHS Direct, it wasn't even his GP, it was his dentist, or whoever used to be his dentist, who had sent him. You see he had not had a check-up for over two years, so he had been automatically taken off the dentist's list. The other dentists in the area were not taking new NHS patients and there was no available emergency dentist, so they had advised him of my expertise if he was in need of painkillers, which he was.

He was pissed off. He didn't want to come to A&E, he wanted his tooth sorted. Luckily, we have an emergency dentist in the area, which our receptionists managed to book him into for the next day.

I felt annoyed with myself for being annoyed with him. It is the system that is at fault and not the patient, but thanks to useless negotiating on behalf of the NHS, the dentistry cover isn't as good as it could be considering the amount of money put into it. People's teeth are getting damaged and because people want an instant fix they come to A&E. It is like so much in society. When the normal health services that a society needs to function are not working too well, then people come to A&E, regardless of whether or not they have an accident or emergency.

Should he have called an ambulance?

Some patients really do try your patience. They abuse the system and it is very hard not be judgmental. I had one tonight – I'll let you decide whether you are happy that your taxes were spent on him.

He was complaining of chest pain, but was well known to us – 14 visits for chest pain in the last year and all on a Saturday or Friday night. Chest pains get seen straight away

– and rightly so – so I asked some questions. He said his pain had gone and then he went. I tried to stop him. I tried to explain that he would benefit from an ECG and that I would like to at least examine him before he left.

'Nah, I have got better things to do,' he said and walked off.

The ambulance men apologised for bringing him. They had to as he had called them complaining of pains in his chest. It is one of those conditions where it is always better to be safe than sorry and come to A&E. However, this man lives just around the corner from the hospital and whenever he is out and gets pissed he calls for a free taxi and lies about chest pain.

What a selfish and thoughtless act, putting other people's lives at risk. One day he will have real chest pain and his past action will have put him at risk as the ambulance crew may not believe him or be tied up with other people like him.

I later found out from another ambulance crew that he had done it again. This time they took him to another hospital 35 miles away from this one and 35.1 miles away from his house. He went berserk when he found out that he was nowhere near home. He demanded a lift home after self-discharging. The ambulance men kindly told him where to go.

I understand that it was an expensive taxi ride home, especially on a Saturday night… we haven't seen him in A&E since. Sometimes you have just got to love your ambulance colleagues. For anyone interested there is a fantastic blog (and book – *Blood, Sweat and Tea*) by an ambulance man – who describes his joys of working in the NHS (http://randomreality. blogware.com).

A different type of health visitor

I knew I was going to enjoy this consultation from the outset. He was 92, looked 72, and had been flirting with the nurses from the moment the ambulance brought him.

'Hello sir. How are you?' I asked.

'You'll have to speak up, I am very deaf,' he responded.

I reassured him that he didn't need to worry as I was very loud. Now that we knew that this wasn't going to be a private conversation, despite closing the curtains around the cubicle (which I used to think made the room soundproof), we started the consultation.

I soon found out that he had chest pain. It sounded like angina – a condition he is known to suffer from. Normally it settles with a spray of a drug called GTN. However, he had first got the pain an hour ago and was still in pain. While my colleague did an ECG, I put in an intravenous line and started some medications to ease the discomfort.

'So what were you doing when the pain came on?' I asked.

'It happened when my health visitor was with me. She was the one who called the ambulance.'

I enquired why he had a health visitor and how often she came round to see him.

'She comes round once every three weeks, just to see how I am and help me… you know.'

I wasn't too sure what he was talking about, but I thought he must have been describing a new government scheme, whereby community matrons visit patients with chronic conditions at home every couple of weeks to check that they are OK. They then liaise with their GP and try and implement plans to keep them out of hospital. I asked him if that was what he meant by a health visitor.

'She isn't organised by the GP. I organised her myself about three years ago. She has been very good to me,' he responded.

Now I was confused. Naive as well, as it turned out! I continued in my questioning.

'So does she help round the house then?'

'No my friend.' He leaned forward and in a theatrical whisper said, 'She comes round to help me ejaculate as I can't really do it myself. It was when she was playing with me that I got the chest pain. It was so bad that she had to stop and call the ambulance.'

'What a bloke', I thought, 'Honest and still enjoying life, and very friendly'. I smiled and in the notes wrote pain started on 'mild exertion'. It is encounters like this that make my job pleasurable.

How targets can hurt patients and staff

In principle, a target to see and sort out patients within 4 hours is a fantastic aspiration. Unfortunately, it is like a lot of targets and reforms – they comply with the law of unintended consequences by creating an unintentional distortion in clinical priority, which impinges on the quality of care we provide.

I don't think Labour has deliberately tried to harm patients care at all, or that it has deliberately tried to piss off NHS staff. I think that its heart is roughly in the right place, it's just that it has implemented some ridiculously stupid NHS reforms without realising the consequences. Do you remember, during the last election, someone complaining to Blair on *Question Time* that they couldn't book follow-up GP appointments? He had no idea that his policy of making all GPs guarantee that they would see people within 48 hours would mean that they would stop making follow-up appointments a week or so in advance. It was an unintended consequence. He was clearly shocked and promised to sort it out.

Well-intentioned cock-ups like this have happened throughout the NHS. Within A&E, we have the 4-hour target – we have 4 hours from when a patient arrives to either discharge them or admit them; 98 per cent of patients need to meet this target. Don't get me wrong; on the whole, the 4-hour target has banged heads together and brought about some good changes to the way we work and treat patients. Patients no longer wait 12 hours to see a doctor for a broken toe and being admitted to hospital has been streamlined. However, unintended consequences do exist and they can be harmful for patients. Let me explain with a couple of examples.

Last week, we were having a very, very busy day. There were massive delays in X-ray and an old lady who had fallen had had to wait 3 hours and 40 minutes to confirm the diagnosis of a fractured hip. She had been given some morphine while waiting for her X-ray, but was still in pain. The clock was ticking – it was 3 hours and 55 minutes since she had come in and the porters were about to be called to take her to the ward. In 5 minutes I could have given her some more morphine. However, it has side-effects such as slowing down the respiration rate (she also had a chest infection, which had caused her to fall in the first place) and nausea. What is just as effective but without the complications of a second morphine injection, is an injection of local anaesthetic into the area around the nerve going to the hip. It numbs the area within 10 minutes, and around 12 hours of pain relief is provided. However, it takes around 15 minutes to do. I told the nurse in charge that I wanted the patient to have the injection and not go to the ward just yet. I was told that she would fail her 4-hour target. This is known as a 'breach'. In these days of targets it is so hard to argue back. If a patient breaches, then the consultants have to 'examine' why. If too many patients 'breach', then the NHS managers come down on the hospital like a ton of bricks and there are potential financial penalties.

But aren't we in the job to provide the best possible care for the patient and not there to worry about targets? No wonder so many nurses and doctors are leaving A&E. They are doing so because they are not allowed to do their job properly – caring and managing patients.

After a 10-minute delay, we all agreed that it was in the patient's interests to give her this injection and the figures were fiddled. (I deliberately do not get involved in this fiddling, because I think we should be producing honest figures so that something gets done rather than just massaging the ego of the Secretary of State for Health.) The department pretended she had left A&E 20 minutes earlier than she had. The figures said that she stayed 3 hours and 59 minutes. It is ridiculous that so much time and energy is spent trying desperately to meet targets, but when we fall short, someone has the job of adjusting the time. I don't blame the A&E department for adjusting the figures. There is such pressure on us to comply with the target that adjustment is seen as acceptable. It means the hospital won't get penalised financially or by a reduction of its 'star performance score' status. By fiddling the figures, it also means that we can concentrate on looking after our patients.

If there hadn't been this target culture, then there wouldn't have been this unnecessary stress and pressure on everyone. Perhaps if targets were used to identify where more resources were needed, rather than to punish failure, patient care might be improved. This time the potential breach was caused by a delay in X-ray (which often occurs). The solution might be to hire an extra radiographer. If this was done – if cash was invested to sort out this problem – then this delay might not occur again. But no, we fiddled the figures so we didn't lose money and hence no one could highlight the problem. And the government could say everything is lovely-jubbly.

Another example was a 16-year-old girl who came in last Thursday. She had been drinking in the joyous surrounding of the local park. (Oh, the joys of the Anglo-Saxon drinking culture.) The ambulance was called because she was unconscious in the street. She needed fluids and a period of observation. At 3 hours and 30 minutes, my colleague reviewed her and determined that although she was now conscious, she was not well enough to go home yet. She needed another few hours to ensure that she didn't still choke on her own vomit, etc. Before the days of targets, she would have stayed in A&E until she was well enough to go home. However, now we could only keep her for 4 hours, although she needed more time. My colleague was then told to refer her to the paediatricians to go and sober up on the kids' ward. This was not appropriate. The paediatricians were busy enough and didn't need to see a patient that my friend knew didn't need their specialist skills, but then there is this bloody 4-hour target. Except in a very few clinical exceptions, we are not allowed to care for someone for longer than this time period. My colleague refused to succumb to the pressure of the nurse managers and did not refer her to the paediatricians and ended up getting a lot of grief for it.

She reviewed the girl 2 hours later. She was fit enough to go home with parental supervision. However, she was discharged about 45 minutes earlier than would have been ideal. The next day the doctor was expecting an interrogation into why she had let someone 'breach' but the figure had been fiddled and the patient was apparently discharged at 3 hours and 59 minutes. Again, I can understand why the figure was fiddled, but if we hadn't fiddled the figures we might have seen the problem and a solution – a properly staffed paediatric A&E observation bed, where patients can be admitted while staying under the A&E team.

Figure fiddling happens everywhere. A recent survey by the British Medical Association and the British Association of Accident and Emergency Medicine showed that 31 per cent of A&E doctors admitted to working in a department where 'data manipulation was used as an additional measure to meet emergency access targets'. In other words, they admitted to working in an A&E where the figures were fiddled.

This is further backed by research from the City University business school that looked at the records of 170 000 A&E attendees and applied 'queuing theory'. The conclusions were reported by lead researcher Professor Les Mayhew, who said:

'The current A&E target is simply not achievable without the employment of dubious management tactics. The government needs to revisit its targets and stop forcing hospitals into a position where they look for ways to creatively report back, rather than actually reducing waiting times for real people.'

When the Department of Health spokesman responds by saying back to the BBC, 'It's absolute nonsense to suggest that the A&E waiting time standard is not being met,' who do you believe?

It is not just the raw data that is manipulated. There are other ways in which 5 hours to you and me means 4 hours to the Department of Health. Examples I have heard from various colleagues throughout the country include:

1. Corridors are re-designated admission wards by the simple application of a curtain rail. As soon as you are admitted to the 'admission ward' the clock stops.
2. Patients are discharged on the computer before they have left the A&E (i.e. before they have got their discharge drugs or similar).
3. As soon as a bed on a ward is allocated to the patient, the patient is transferred to that bed on the computer, regardless of whether they have to wait an hour for the porters to take them to it.
4. Patients can be admitted by computer to an A&E ward (and not breach) but physically not move because there are a lot more beds on the computer than there are in real life.
5. The time it takes from the ambulance bringing a patient in to being logged onto the computer can take up to

30 minutes longer if there are no nurses to meet the ambulance. The clock starts ticking when we are ready and when the receptionist has had her cup of tea, NOT when you arrive.

6. If a patient has been referred by a GP, they don't come to A&E anymore, but to an admission ward. As they are technically admitted, there is no target for how quickly they get seen and so they can often languish for hours before seeing a doctor.

7. Patients for whom A&E doctors have asked for a review by a specialist can get admitted to a ward regardless of whether the specialist has seen them or not and regardless of whether they actually need to come in or not. Once admitted to a ward they can stay there for ages without being seen by the specialist as they are no longer in A&E and so cannot breach.

8. Originally, there were specific days when the 4-hour rules were being assessed. On that day, the hospitals would cancel elective operations so that there were spare beds and employed loads of extra locum doctors and nurses to make it look as if the hospital was more efficient than it really was.

So, as you can see, hospitals feel compelled to massage their figures. The target was brought in for the right reason and initially did a very good job. But we need clinicians to make the priorities, not politicians. If the government is going to insist on targets, then let's make some sensible ones such as all urgently triaged patients to be seen within 5 minutes of arrival. Or how about patients being able to expect a bed 30 minutes after they have been fully treated in A&E, etc? These targets may not be as glamorous to tell voters about, but they might actually improve care without distorting priorities.

The reason I moan so much about this is that what was once a tool to improve A&E is now damaging patient care and doctors' and nurses' sanities. I just hope a politician or two reads these words and does something about it other than claim that what we are saying is just 'nonsense'.

At work on New Year's Eve

I am writing this on New Years Day. Last night I was at work and it was absolute hell. The A&E looked like a war zone – police restraining aggressive drunks, teenagers vomiting and crying and overworked staff acting as bouncers. I can only assume that the managers thought that someone might fiddle figures for the night and so didn't bother to employ any extra staff despite knowing how busy it was going to be. I was knackered by the end of the shift and was pissed off with some of the patients' attitudes, but in all honesty, I quite enjoyed myself.

But I can hardly blame the new drinking laws. I started my shift at 9 p.m. and the drunks were already there. The first was quite a nice lad of about 17. He had fallen asleep in the street and someone had called an ambulance because he had wet himself and was vomiting.

'So what happened?' I asked.

'You tell me,' he retorted.

'No. I asked first. What happened?' I countered.

'Don't know mate. Been larging it,' he said in his irritatingly pretend street speak accent – posh but with a touch of Estuary English.

'It says on the notes from the nurse that you have been drinking. That can't be true as you are under 18 and so surely can't have been drinking. What actually happened?' I mocked.

'Nah mate, I gone massive. I am quality,' he retorted in Mockney.

Luckily, I listen to Radio One, so I sort of understood what he had said.

'So how have you gone massive mate?' I enquired.

'Vodka mate. Bottle of vodka – down in 1 hour. Larging it. So what am I doing here?'

I explained that an ambulance had been called for him as he was so drunk.

'That is quality. Coming to hospital 'cos so drunk. Quality.'

I asked some questions to check that he was OK and had suffered no ill-effects from his night's drinking. I asked him if he thought a bottle of vodka was really that sensible for a 17-year-old's liver.

'I can do it because I am so f**king hard. I am hard as nails me.'

'Right… so hard you end up vomiting all night and pissing yourself so that your mummy had to collect you at 10 p.m.? Yep, hard, aren't you? Well done mate.'

I called in his mother, and as soon as he was able to walk without falling over, he went home. Except that that wasn't all he had to say for himself. While waiting for his mum, every couple of minutes he would call out to one of the nurses.

'Oi! Beautiful! I am quality – do you want to come home with me?'

He was harmless but irritating after a while.

The next case was a 14-year-old girl. The ambulance called ahead to say they were blue lighting her in as she was completely unconscious. The nurse and junior doctor tried to wake her up and couldn't. I got a call on the intercom.

I walked in and initially failed as well. If she was truly unconscious then we might have to intubate her (i.e. put her to sleep and take over her breathing) so that she wouldn't choke to death on her own vomit, which I was currently sucking out of her mouth (with a suction tube). Then I tried a 'registrar's trapezius squeeze'. (Basically, you squeeze as hard as possible on the bit of muscle between the neck and shoulder, then carry on squeezing until they wake up.) She did wake up – very quickly. I checked that she hadn't hit her head or taken any drugs, asked the senior nurse to put in an intravenous cannula, watch for more vomiting, and give her some fluids.

Giving fluids to someone who is drunk is a little controversial. We spend tax-payers' money helping them to sober up and not get as bad a hangover which may positively reinforce their A&E-seeking behaviour after drinking. This can't be good, but I am still a believer in giving them lots of fluids when people are drunk because it helps to get rid of them more quickly. It helps them sober up, and also they soon wake up needing to go to the toilet. Sometimes it backfires and they end up losing full control of their now full bladder – but the risk is worth taking as it is so effective in aiding appropriate discharges.

I explained to the girl's mum what was happening and why we were giving her daughter fluids. We put the girl on her side and left her where we could watch her closely. We also gave her little sister, who had to enjoy her New Year's Eve watching her big sister vomit, a chair and a blanket to cuddle into.

After 3 hours and 59 minutes the girl was sober enough to go home with her mum, who was furious with her daughter. As I came to see her, her mum was in the middle of telling her off.

'This is the second time you have done this now. You have ruined your New Year and everyone's else's, you selfish girl,' I heard her say. I introduced myself to the young girl and checked she was OK. I then said she was free to go but before that I wanted give her some useful patient education.

'You could have died you know – you are only 14. Don't be so dangerous in future.'

She looked at the floor.

'Do you want me to tell her off?' I asked her mum.

'Please do,' she said.

'I have seen loads of people ruin their lives by binge drinking. You have been so stupid. We had to suck out the vomit from your mouth. Do you realise that? Do you? You could have had the vomit go into your lungs and then you wouldn't have been able to breathe properly. You could have died, and in that state anybody could have done anything to you and you wouldn't have known. Don't be so stupid again and drink with some self respect.'

Her mother seemed suitably pleased with me. But I hadn't yet finished.

'You have also stopped me seeing really sick people who needed my help. The elderly lady in cubicle 5 had to wait an extra 30 minutes for me to give her pain killers for her broken leg because of your selfish stupidity.'

Her mum seemed very pleased with my chastising abilities, but then said, through gritted teeth, 'You wait till you get home and then you'll get a proper telling off.' I felt sorry for the girl: I obviously had not been stern enough!

There are probably some trust guidelines saying that my attitude to this patient was probably not appropriate – I didn't treat her in a holistic way and I didn't communicate in a way appropriate to understanding her cultural needs (i.e. she was an Anglo-Saxon who culturally needed to binge drink). A lot of doctors, who are worried about having to be politically correct, may not have acted in that way for fear of being complained about. But I think that we should be complained about if we *don't* try and educate patients on harm prevention. We need them to know the danger of their behaviour and it has been shown that short blasts from A&E doctors can make a difference. It is also quite enjoyable for us, but that is not the point. If I really wanted to go into a job so I could tell off teenagers, I would have gone into teaching. But then all my teacher friends say that if they really wanted to go into a job where they could tell off teenagers, then they would have been A&E doctors. Anyway my fears that I had gone a bit over the top subsided when in the morning, her mum brought round a thank you letter and a box of chocolates. I have never been thanked so kindly for being so forthright to someone's offspring before.

The effects of drinking continued. Luckily, as it got later in the evening, the patients generally got a little older. Unfortunately, they also got a little more abusive as their waits to see me increased. There was a lot of drinking going on – mostly on empty stomachs but largely on empty heads as well

– a particularly dangerous combination. The only difference from New Year's Eve in the days before liberal drinking laws is that now cases of alcohol intoxication continue from 8 p.m. to 6 a.m.

The thing to remember is that these patients do need proper medical care – in fact they often need even better attention than sober patients as it is easy to miss injuries when someone is drunk. More seriously, it is easy to misdiagnose an unconscious patient as someone being drunk, when in fact they have had a serious head injury. I left work absolutely exhausted, but with a thought. If only we could videotape these patients and then show them what fools they made of themselves...

Why bother coming?

It's a Sunday. The weather is beautiful. There are hills to walk up, football matches to watch, women/men to chat up, beer to drink and the seaside is only an hour's drive away. You are young and healthy, with money in your back pocket – the world is your oyster. Lastminute.com is offering you 12 hours in New York for £3, the cinema has a new movie on; you have a new horny girlfriend who has lost her rabbit. You could do anything. So why on earth do you sit in A&E for 5 hours (sorry, Mrs Hewitt, 3 hours and 59 minutes on the computer), for me to see you and say there is nothing wrong with you? Look, go to your GP if you are worried about non-urgent things and next time you come, read the sign outside – ACCIDENT AND EMERGENCY DEPARTMENT.

Some examples from the last few days:

1. 8-year-old kid at school. Fell over and grazed his knee. Played football for 30 minutes after injury before the bleeding became too noticeable. His school was not happy to take the responsibility to wash the graze and give him a paracetamol. So the poor kid waited 4 hours and 30 minutes (whoops… 3 hours and 59 minutes to you, Mrs Secretary of State for Health) to see a nurse to have it cleaned and bandaged. If the kid had just had a teacher who was legally allowed to show common sense, he could have been at school having fun and perhaps learning something, as opposed to sitting in the waiting room all day.

2. 50-year-old man: 'Doctor, I went to bed and woke up and felt scared and so called an ambulance.' He was having a nightmare. Now, I am not annoyed with him, just the lack of mental health support in the community, which can look after patients with his type of condition.

3. Man with chronic hip pain – no worse – had it for two years. The GP he likes is on holiday, so came to us instead. Needs a new hip, but doesn't need to come to A&E. Poor bloke, not annoyed with him, but more at the system for allowing waiting lists of eight months for hip operations. (N.B. Clever statistics would show that he has only been waiting four months for the hip, but he waited four months to see the orthopaedic surgeon to tell him that he needs an operation. In the real world that is an eight-month wait. In NHS world, it is four months. However, that is still much better than in the days of the Tories ruining the NHS. Now

at least the waiting lists are coming down quickly – even if they have done it in a very expensive and divisive way.)

4. 28-year-old man – pain in his foot for three days after playing football. No obvious injury and has been able to run on it but as it was still sore this morning, he called an ambulance. Not taken any analgesia. Well, if he had, it might not hurt so much. He demanded an X-ray; I asked why he had called an ambulance. He said he paid his 'f**king taxes to get X-rays when he wanted one', but didn't answer my ambulance question. I reminded him that he paid his taxes so that I could decide if I would X-ray him. He went on about patient choice to call an ambulance and choice of getting an X-ray. I had to listen to his twaddle and be polite. It was hard. I wish there was a campaign for doctor choice as well as patient choice. I would have chosen to tell him where to go. Instead, I was polite and moaned about him when I got home from work.

There are loads more. People will not take responsibility for themselves or others. Some are just selfish, others just have mental health issues and the community services are not in place. Some just don't go to their GP for one reason or another. In the end, there is no inappropriate A&E attendee, just someone who doesn't know what the alternatives are (and when they should be used), or who lives in an area where the alternatives are not properly resourced.

ℒ I am so glad I am tired

Last night I went to bed at 10 p.m. My wife was not well at all, high temperature, coughing and sneezing and lethargy – Man 'flu, I diagnosed, and so I agreed to look after our non-sleeping child all night. I was nervous and the anticipation of being awakened stopped me falling asleep. I resorted to desperate measures – I started reading the *British Medical Journal*: 30 seconds later, I was out like a light.

Two hours later the crying started. Back to sleep, and then up again at 2 a.m., then 4 a.m. and then 5.30 a.m. I wish I could invent a cure for colic and teething – something more ethical than ear plugs. But alas no... So, off to work at 7.30 a.m. and I was exhausted. I believe that the bastard who invented the term 'sleeps like a baby' never met anyone under five.

I arrived as the red phone went off. Information from the ambulance crew – paediatric arrest. Patient, six months, mottled and blue on arrival. The senior nurse called the paediatric resuscitation team down, but we all knew the probable outcome: this was a cot death and we were going to be going through the motions just in case and also to help the long-term grieving process.

The child came in with mother screaming. The thing I noticed was that he had the cutest little blue socks on which were the same colour as his skin. Our initial expectations were correct. We had all agreed our jobs, with the paediatric registrar being in charge of us all. My job was to get an interosseous line in (this is where a needle is quickly inserted into baby's leg bone as a very quick way to give fluid and drugs – you do this when they are so ill they have no visible blood vessels). I got on with my job, but felt sick. I wasn't in charge and could just concentrate on my job. Somehow I felt very detached from the whole situation. All the voices seemed distant. The mum's cry was audible, as was the counting of the cardiac compressions, but it all felt surreal. I can't explain why I felt like this but I did. I pushed the needle a little harder and felt the pop of the needle going through the baby's bone. It was a huge sense of relief that I had done the part I was supposed to do. I attached the needle to fluids and gave drugs that others had drawn up.

The drugs were not helping – nothing was. We were keeping his blood pumping with the compressions and the anaesthetist was breathing for him – but he was dead and had been for a long time. We all knew it but nobody wanted to give up. Nobody wanted to stay 'Stop' in front of mum.

It felt like fruitless cruelty, but I rationalised it by knowing that the child would feel nothing and the grief would perhaps be easier in the long run for mum and dad if they knew we had tried everything.

I wanted to say 'Stop' but my colleague in charge murmured a suggestion of doubling the usual adrenaline dose – no-one really thought it would work, but no one said so. It is much easier to stop resuscitating an elderly adult than a child. No one wants to be the first to say stop. After about 15 minutes, one of the senior nurses first brought up stopping. No-one really responded – but a general agreement was made to continue for another cycle (2 minutes)

But then, thankfully, the (right) decision was taken out of our hands. 'Please stop… Stop, STOP. STOP. He's dead… My baby is dead.' We all looked at each other, nodded and stopped.

The barbaric-looking lines and tubes were removed and the senior nurse wrapped him in a blanket. He picked him up and took him to mum. She held him and sobbed, and sobbed and sobbed… and then started speaking to him, 'I am so sorry I let you down today. I'll make it up to you. Tomorrow, we can go to the zoo and see all those animals you like.'

At this point I couldn't stay in the resuscitation room any longer. The consultant paediatrician was coming in from home to talk with the mother about what had happened. I was so glad it wasn't my job, because all I wanted to do was cry and have a cup of tea.

I made the tea and went to calm my nerves for a few minutes. I was soon interrupted by one of the new nurse managers who came and found me and barked an order, 'The bloke in cubicle three needs to be seen now or he is going to breach his 4-hour target,' he said. I couldn't believe it. I had just been part of a failed resuscitation of a child and all he cared about was some poxy figure. 'I couldn't care less,' I wanted to scream. Unfortunately, all I ended up muttering was 'I'll be there in a minute.' How I hate myself when that happens.

The senior nurse, who had been at the failed resuscitation, came and found me, gave me a hug and said, 'Have your tea. Sod the pointless figures… someone can always fiddle them.'

I smiled, happy that the vast majority of nurses have kept their sanity despite the government interference, and went to my next job: a man who had called an ambulance for a painful shoulder which he had for 4 years… ah, the joys of working in A&E…

By the end of my shift, I was exhausted. But I was so, so glad I was tired – my child had kept me up all night. That other kid's mum and dad had had an undisturbed night's sleep. That little boy wouldn't have made a sound for the last few hours.

…What a shit start to the day.

People we refer to

The A&E doctors often refer to specialist doctors and other health-care professionals. Listed below are a few of the people we work with and what they do. (*This is all tongue-in-cheek and if I offend anyone, then I am truly sorry.*)

Radiologists – doctors who specialise in looking at X-rays and scans. Older ones specialise in explaining why the test you want to do is not justified, younger ones specialise in not only doing the test, but then putting various tubes in to the patient while they are having the test. Never call them radiographers – apparently they get upset.

Plastic surgeons – as consultants they spend a lot of their time making money out of people with low self-esteem. As trainees they spend a lot of their time treating burn victims and nasty hand injuries.

Respiratory specialists – know a lot about chests, tuberculosis (TB) and asthma. Like to titter when they say to patients 'big breaths'. (If anyone says this to you, do NOT say 'well thank you doctor!' and play with your hair.)

Cardiologists – experts on knowing lots about the heart. They are also experts on making sure that you know that they know a lot about the heart. They like the phrase 'A stent in time, saves nine!' The last breed of doctors to not realise that wearing a bow tie makes them look like an idiot.

Junior surgeons – cavalier with their approach to cutting.

Senior surgeons – cavalier with their approach to putting.

Gynaecologists – the Heineken of all doctors. Can reach the parts that others can't.

Acute medical doctors – look after a very similar type of patients to A&E doctors with a similar approach; but have got longer than 4 hours to play with.

General medical doctors – look after patients with 'medical' conditions (e.g. heart attacks, strokes, heart failure, pneumonia). Like to organise a lot of tests – the more expensive the better.

Paediatricians – look after little kids. Always happy. Colourful ties. Generally nice.

Orthopaedic surgeons (orthopods) – known as the carpenters of the medical world through their mending of bones and replacing of joints. They take pride in knowing as little medicine as possible. They are the butt of medical doctors' jokes – replace the word 'blonde/Irish' with the word 'orthopod' and the joke is usually funny to doctors. Favourite ortho jokes include:

– How many orthopods does it take to change a light bulb? One: referral to the medics, 'darkness, query cause?'

– What is the definition of a double-blind trial? Two orthopods looking at an ECG. – What is the difference between an orthopaedic surgeon and a carpenter? The carpenter knows more than one antibiotic, etc., etc.

Rheumatologists – give you tablets for your arthritis. When they stop working, send you to the orthopods.

Psychiatrists – don't like people saying 'You should have your head examining if you want to see a psychiatrist.' A lot of their time in A&E is for risk assessment for depressed patients; a small proportion of their time is for truly floridly psychotic patients. Generally poor taste in clothes – sandals and tweed. Use phrases such as 'erotic counter transference', when trying to explain that they thought their last patient was quite fit (in the attractive, not necessarily athletic sense).

Anaesthetists – put people to sleep for surgery, usually by drugs but sometimes by conversation. Very useful when we have very sick patients as they can put in central lines (large intravenous lines through which fluids, blood and drugs can be given quickly) and take over their breathing when patients are struggling. More and more A&E doctors are learning these skills too. So, in the future, we may have to call for these doctors' help less and less. They can therefore spend more time concentrating on their specialist subjects – sudoku and crosswords at the local independent treatment centre.

Renal doctors – look after patients who have damaged kidneys. Highly intelligent, but can be a little dull.

Understand glomerulonephritis and cANCA. (see Glossary, p.291). Be wary of dialysis specialists. They get offended easily, so don't take the piss out of them. It's their job to do that to their patients

Geriatricians – unsung heroes of the NHS. See massive amounts of patients and act in pragmatic way – by not treating each sign and symptom but the patient. Sometimes difficult to tell the doctor from the patient.

Oncologists – sung heroes of the NHS. Fair enough, though, they do a good job.

Palliative care doctors – treat terminal patients.

Aviation doctors – treat patients in terminals.

Midwives – they deliver babies and us from evil. Don't mess or answer back. Ever!

Dermatologists – If you are able to refer to one of these as an emergency, you work in a big teaching hospital. They look at rashes and give them a Latin name to look clever and then prescribe steroids

Ophthalmologists – eye specialists. Could replace their on-call service with an automated answer message. 'Press 1 for me to say give chloramphenicol ointment and I will see them in the morning', press 2 for me to say give chloramphenicol and review in two days time', etc.

Urologists – willie doctors. They love them – short ones, big ones, thin ones, long ones, fractured ones, infected ones, bent ones, lacerated ones… any type – they will have them. Also look after kidney stones and the prostate gland and erectile dysfunction – which isn't an A&E condition. Please remember that I do not give

Viagra from A&E, so don't come and ask for it... even if she is really fit and you haven't had any for years. And no, I will not call a urologist to prescribe it for you either. Not getting a hard-on is not an accident or emergency condition. Go to your GP... Sorry, I just remembered a patient who made me irate about six months ago.

So there you have it. Now when you hear a doctor say that they are going to refer you to a so-and-so doctor, you will know what to expect.

Why patients are more important than budgets

I saw a 76-year-old gentleman yesterday. The poor man had had a stroke. He had very severe weakness down his left side. Once the stroke has already occurred, there is little that can be done initially for the patient (although at some hospitals, strokes are being treated like heart attacks and clot-busting drugs are given). Generally, though, it is more about long-term rehabilitation and preventing further strokes.

When I looked at the A&E notes from exactly four weeks ago, I noticed that he had come in with a TIA (transient ischaemic attack) – often called a 'mini' or 'warning' stroke. He had had 10 minutes of arm weakness which had resolved. Quite rightly, the doctor who had examined him had ascertained that it had resolved and he could go home. The A&E doctor wanted to refer him to a rapid access 'TIA/stroke prevention' clinic. In these clinics, a specialist tries to reduce the chance of a stroke happening. Patients get an urgent CT (computed tomography) brain scan and a scan on the neck (in case there is a blocked artery which may need an operation), not to mention getting started on the necessary drugs to prevent further strokes such as aspirin. If he had been referred, this would have been excellent A&E treatment. A letter to the GP would have let them know what was going on. The problem was that he was not referred to the clinic. Owing to the financing arrangements of hospitals and GPs, we are encouraged not to make direct referrals but to refer the patient back to their GP for them to make the referral to the clinic. The reason for this is purely arbitrary accounting rules. Although the cost is all borne by the NHS, if the referral comes from the GP, it comes from a different pot and the hospital can then be paid by the PCT (primary care trust). Dull accountancy facts, but important for this patient.

The waste of time is the thing that annoys me (for the patient, not just the GP). The patient couldn't see the GP over the weekend and then, when he booked an appointment, he didn't tell the receptionist it was urgent and asked to see his regular GP who only worked two days a week and was on holiday. As a result, he had to wait till the following Tuesday – a delay of 10 days so far. The referral was then promptly made, but he had not yet been seen in clinic by the time he came back to A&E. This is despite evidence-based medicine advocating that these patients are seen in clinic within two weeks of a warning stroke. It is upsetting that at courses and medical school we learn the gold standard of care but then often end up only being able to provide a silver or bronze quality of care because of local guidelines, management structures or rationing of resources.

I am not saying that this delay in being seen in clinic was the cause of his stroke, but if A&E could have referred him to the clinic, he might have had an operation and the stroke could possibly have been prevented. But no, the NHS has become disjointed, with separate parts working independently of each other without the cooperation that used to be present. Accountancy rules ruled over clinical care.

Sadly, this is just one example. So that hospitals can earn money when patients are seen in clinic, A&E doctors refer fewer and fewer patients to specialist clinics. Everything must go through GPs now. This is sensible for conditions that may be chronic and for which the GPs may have already organised various tests, but for new conditions these rules are madness. It is an inefficient use of GP time and a waste of resources.

Accountancy rules run the NHS and not common sense. In some hospitals, even consultants, who see patients in outpatient departments at the GP's request and want an opinion from another specialist before making final treatment judgments, have to refer them back to their GP for the GP to refer on. If this isn't done, then apparently the hospital won't get paid for the cost of the second opinion.

So why are these rules in place? Part of the logic of this is also to do with the new concept of patient choice and the involvement of the private sector. The government thinks that it can drive up standards and save money by making GPs the purse holders to the NHS. 'Payment by results' is the term it is using to mean that primary care trusts via your GP pay for 'episodes of care'. This is why the referrals need to come *from* your GP and not a hospital doctor (who in fact may know a lot more about your current problem because they have been dealing with you.) The GPs can now refer you to your local hospital or a local private treatment centre, depending on patient preference. This is OK in principle but most patients, if they had the choice, would choose a local well-run hospital where profit was not a concern. What is happening is that money is being taken out of hospitals and spent on private companies. The hospitals are suffering as a result and are starting to have to compete against these private treatment centres.

Some hospitals will be good at one thing and charge a cheaper rate and get the business. Others will not be so good and then lose business. So, in the future, your local hospital may not have all the necessary services. For example, your local knee surgeon may have been made redundant and had to move 70 miles away to the local 'knee specialist hospital'. This is fine for elective operations but what happens if you are in a car accident and your knee is damaged? Now that there is no longer an experienced knee surgeon working at your local hospital you either have to travel miles to a 'centre of excellence' or possibly receive substandard care locally. This is the logical end result of current government thinking.

When the government was implementing these changes I don't think that they thought through the effects that these changes would have on emergency-care patients. An unintended consequence of payment by results and patient choice is services being damaged at the local hospitals as well as referrals to clinics being delayed. If the government truly wants patient choice then let patients have what they are asking for: properly run local hospitals where care comes before accountancy rules and regulations.

♫ An occupational hazard

A teenager would sometimes love my job, but there are hazards. It was 7.30 a.m. and the last patient before I finished, and I was looking forward to some scrambled eggs in the canteen. He had come in with a nasty abscess on his buttock. He needed it incised and drained. I put a scalpel in the abscess and squeezed. Pus upon pus squeezed out. I gave it one last squeeze and then disaster struck. The pus squirted straight in my face. Egg-like Staph. infection all over my right cheek and glasses. I remained professional, finished the minor operation, then left my nurse colleague to finish off dressing the wound and went to wash my face thoroughly. As I found the sink and disinfectant, my colleague, who was starting his shift, saw what had had happened and reminded me of the time when this happened to him about a month ago. Except that his mouth was open at the time and he wasn't wearing any glasses.

Feeling a bit sick, I decided to give scrambled eggs a miss this morning and went to sleep without breakfast, but after a very long shower.

♫ I don't understand some patients

Last night I saw a patient who was having unstable angina. He needed drugs to relieve the pain and treat the condition, but despite about an hour of persuasion he refused to let me put a needle into his arm, and give him the drugs. He explained that he did not believe in western medicine and therefore refused my drugs. Why he came to A&E in that case was beyond me, but it was really difficult seeing a man whom I could have so easily helped sit there in agony. However, patients (quite rightly) have a right to decide what treatment they will or will not accept. It's just that I did not understand why he came if he was going to refuse treatment.

The case reminded me of another man I had seen a few weeks ago with a dislocated shoulder. I needed to give him morphine for pain relief but he refused an intravenous cannula because he was scared of needles. Normally, a couple of minutes persuasion and they will agree to it; but not him. The thing that confused me on this occasion was, if he was so scared of needles, how come he had so many tattoos?

A trip round A&E

When patients come to A&E, they only see the small bit of A&E that they are in. This quick guide tells you a little about what is in an A&E department so, if you can't see things going on, then at least you may know where the doctors and nurses are and what they might be doing.

Let's start the tour at the front entrance. It is often a very flash and expensively done-up area of the A&E department. You may find a 'mission statement' on the wall. These are usually 'management speak' rubbish about striving for optimal health in a holistic way, while encompassing your disabilities and understanding your cultural sensitivities, blah, blah, blah. If you have a half-hour wait read it. If you have a 3-hour wait to be seen, kill some time and try and translate it into English.

Alternative things you could read are adverts for 'no-win, no-fee' solicitors and the in-house hospital glossy magazine: reading either is bad for your blood pressure.

So, you walk in and get to the reception area. Depending on where you live, there will either be a security guard near by and bullet-proof glass, or a vase and some flowers.

After you have booked in, you go to the triage nurse. They have a nice room, with lots of bandages and splints, etc., and they decide how sick you actually are and therefore who you are going to see and where. You can become a 'majors patient', because they think that you may need a bed to lie on, or a 'minors patient', where you will get a seat in a waiting room, or, if they think you might die because you are so unwell, you will get sent to the resuscitation room. The same process of triage happens if you come by ambulance but is not done in the triage room, but in the main part of the A&E. Unless you have been sent direct by your GP to one of the specialist doctors you will see an A&E doctor in one of those three areas. However, in a few cases the triage nurse may think it appropriate for a specialist doctor to see you straight away (e.g. if you are very pregnant) and may send you straight to the ward.

Recently, changes have meant that if your condition is minor, the triage nurse may redirect you to your GP or get an emergency nurse practitioner (ENP) to see you. They may even discharge you themselves. These triage nurses have done extra training to be called SMINTS (senior minor injury nurse triage). They are also called 'See and Treat', often nicknamed 'See, Treat and Street' them.

Minors is a less high-tech part of A&E. There are plaster trolleys lying around and lots of bandages. Minors is a very poor name. It may be a minor injury that you have, but it could be very significant to your quality of life. It is also quite demeaning to patients to say they are a minor case. But anyway...

Down the corridor from minors is usually the Radiology department, where they do X-rays, etc. In minors, you can often hear screams as minor fractures are relocated here and local anaesthetic injected. Not that exciting.

Majors is where you see elderly patients who have collapsed due to an unknown cause. You also see patient with chest pains. Apparently, other patients get seen there, but I don't seem to see many others. We do blood tests here and send them for scans and X-rays if necessary. From here we can send our patients to one of five places. 'Home' and the 'mortuary' are self explanatory (although should never be mixed up). If they have a condition which just needs observation – i.e. a head injury – they can be sent to the A&E overnight ward, if your hospital is lucky enough to have one, which is usually situated somewhere near the A&E department. If your condition means that you will need longer than 4 hours before we can decide whether you need admission or not you may get sent to a CDU ward (CDU stands for clinical decision unit – not the 'can't decide unit'). Please note, if you need hospital admission you shouldn't be sent to the A&E ward or CDU ward – you may go there only if there is nowhere else to send you. Lastly, you can be sent to a normal ward, if the doctors think you need admission. Very rarely do you get sent from A&E to the appropriate specialist ward. More often, you go to the MAU (Medical Admissions Unit), where they might send you for a short stay to be further assessed before going to the appropriate specialist ward.

At any stage, the A&E doctor may ask a specialist doctor to review the patient, who may or may not admit them to a hospital bed. The doctor who decides if you need admission is initially the A&E doctor but that plan may be changed by the specialist doctor. It is confusing, but trust me when I say I am trying to simplify it!

The final place you may go is the resuscitation room – Resus. This is the high-tech bit of A&E. Lots of machines go beep here. There is the equipment to put people to sleep and defibrillators to restart their hearts. I find this the most relaxing part of A&E as you don't get constantly disturbed by trivia and you always get a nurse allocated to work with you. From here, the very sickest patients often go direct to the mortuary, via the viewing/grieving room. However, if they are lucky they also can go to ICU from here, or, once stabilised, back into A&E and then to a ward. The traumas and cardiac arrests are all seen here and there are often many doctors involved in these patients' care as we call the Resus and trauma teams down from the wards to help the A&E doctors (teams are composed of the on-call doctors for that day from specialties such as Anaesthetics, Medicine, Surgery and Orthopaedics – depending on the type of call put out. Again, don't get the calls mixed up as you really don't want an orthopaedic doctor at a cardiac arrest call).

There are lots of other bits to A&E that you probably won't see: the offices – usually far too many of them; the store rooms (where, contrary to popular belief, there is very little 'action'); stock cupboards and the utility rooms where bodily fluids are cleared away. Finally there is a coffee room and a seminar room. To me it all feels strangely like home.

A&E Room 101

I don't know if you have heard of *Room 101*. It is a vaguely amusing programme with Paul Merton as the host, where guests come along and say what they would eradicate from society to make their life a better place – for example, parking attendants, men wearing sarongs, Simon Cowell-inspired boy bands, Simon Cowell, etc.

I have been thinking that if I could, I would like to be able to go on *Room 101*. I would pick the things I could get rid of in society to make my life at work easier (i.e. make there be fewer accidents), so I can spend less time seeing patients and more time flirting with the nurses.

I have compiled a list – I have called it the A&E Room 101:

1. Lawn bowls – a surprise choice coming at number 1. The number of little old ladies coming in with a fractured hip after tripping on a bowls ball is ridiculous... And the stress of the game! I have seen two heart attacks induced by the high-pressure situations of the inter-village summer lawn competition. Why can't these people play a less dangerous sport? I have never seen anyone over 70 with a rugby injury or a hang-gliding injury. So come on you health and safety managers. Let's ban bowls.

2. Wonderbra adverts – in at 2 this is possibly another surprise choice – sexy roadside advertising – especially those 'Hello boys!' Wonderbra adverts with the fit girl. When that advert was around, I used

to dread coming to work. I would have a number of conversations similar to this one : 'Yeah. I was just driving to work and I got distracted by that advert of the fit bird with her big tits covered by a Wonderbra. Anyway I had to have a look, know what I mean. Just as my head was in the opposite direction to the way my car was going, I crashed into a wall. So here I am – my arm is broke.'

3. 4 × 4 (Chelsea tractors), especially the ones with bull bars – 4 x 4s are designed for muddy terrains; bull bars are designed for hitting bulls. However, these eco-friendly 'Chelsea-ites' don't realise this. They drive in areas that are surfaced with tarmac, with lots of kids running around – there are very few bulls. So when the car hits a kid (instead of a bull), it does what it is designed for and injures the kid (instead of a bull) while protecting the car from being damaged. If you need a 4 x 4 because of where you live, then fair enough. But otherwise think about other people's safety before going out on the school run.

4. Motorised mini scooters – why are they on our streets and estates? They are possibly the most dangerous things I have ever seen. They are tiny bikes that go very fast and you crouch on them. A lot of people fall off. Quite a few get really nasty injuries. They were sold with the proviso that they were not toys and were only to be used in private estates. The people that sold them knew that the people who bought them would live on estates where ponies are trainers and butlers are a type of cigarette. Were they more interested in

profit than public safety? I wonder. Please don't buy one for your kids. They really are dangerous.

5. Excessive outdoor Christmas decorations – apart from being aesthetically Chavy, they cause problems for two reasons: (a) people fall off roofs and get electrocuted while putting them up and (b) people drive past them and look at them saying 'what is that Chavy monstrosity?', and fail to notice the car in front until it too late.

6. Skateboards – but only in the over-18s. When I was at junior school, I used to play on one and would occasionally fall off. I once broke my wrist because of it, but it was an accepted occupational hazard of being a kid. However, there is no excuse for anyone over 18 to play with a skateboard. Do you know how stupid you look doing it, especially when you fall off and have to come to A&E? Leave adults to drink and smoke, and leave kids to play on skateboards. The same applies to BMX bikes. As a public education measure, even if it is not cool, please get your kids to wear a helmet and knee and elbow pads. It would mean I would dread working the school holiday days that little bit less.

7. *JackAss* – the hit TV show and film. A group of pain-resistant Americans do stupidly dangerous stuff and then film it. Luckily, they say at the beginning that these are performed by stunt actors and that kids shouldn't copy them – well, that works, doesn't it? That'll stop them – they think 'Oh no I won't try and imitate these cool people; I'll go and play chess with

Tarquin now.' A couple of years ago I had a spate of kids dive-bombing out of a tree while screaming 'JACKASS'. They often went through a bush onto the ground below, into A&E via an ambulance and then onto theatre via the CT scanner. I am dreading the new film coming out.

8. Ineffective safety warnings – companies are so worried that they are going to get sued nowadays that they put ridiculous disclaimers everywhere. So many, in fact, that they start to become ineffective. For example, last week I had a patient with an anaphylactic reaction to nuts. She had a known allergy, but says she now ignores all disclaimers for 'may contain nuts or nut extracts or made in a factory where nuts are used or once been within a 50-mile radius of a nut' otherwise she would have nothing to eat. They are now put on everything for fear of being sued and it is completely uninformative, so she ignores them all. One thing I don't object to, and others do, are stupid warnings. For example: KP nuts, WARNING. MAY CONTAIN NUTS. McDonalds coffee, WARNING. CONTENTS ARE HOT AND MAY SCALD. I think these signs save the lives of a particular subgroup of people who often attend A&E and I thank the companies for their corporate responsibility.

9. The new ethos of excessive risk management and risk avoidance – schools and clubs are scared to take their kids on trips for fear of the consequences of an accident. Things have become so rigid in society that people are going against the excessive bureaucracy

and doing the most bizarre and dangerous sports and challenges – kite surfing, grass tobogganing and such like. It is two fingers to the no-risk culture and gets their adrenaline pumping... and when they have their horrendous accident and come to A&E, it gets me injecting adrenaline into them.

How to be a good patient

The government wants to increase patient choice. I want to increase doctor choice. I want a system where we choose and book and decide which patients we are going to see; depending on how 'good' they will be as a patient. It will never happen. Instead, just for my own amusement, I have compiled a list of qualities that make you a good patient to see in A&E.

1. Have an accident.
2. ...or an emergency.
3. Always, always, unless you fulfil criteria 1 or 2, go to your GP first. They get paid a lot more than me.
4. ...Even if you don't like bothering them.
5. ...Even if you have to wait 2 hours for an appointment.
6. See point 3 again just to make sure you remember it.
7. Don't come just because your no-win, no-fee, no self-respect lawyer has told you to come.
8. If you have had a bad back/knee/ankle for more than 2 days, try pain killers before coming to see me.
9. Please bring a list of the pills you take. Ridiculously, we haven't got access to GPs' computer records and so,

no, I don't know what you are on. It also takes about 4 hours to get your hospital records, so don't say 'You must have a list in the files.' Also, please note that there are thousands of little white pills and even if it does taste bitter, it doesn't help me pinpoint exactly what you are taking.

10. Don't just come for a chat because you are lonely. Go to the pub or your GP.

11. Don't call an ambulance because you don't want to spend money on a taxi (they are there for people who need them).

12. …or because you think it will get you seen quicker – it doesn't.

13. Don't remind me that you have to be seen and discharged within 4 hours – I know, but I am not sitting on my arse, I might just be seeing someone sicker than you who met the criteria in points 1 and 2.

14. If you must mention the '4-hour rule' (see point 13) at least get the facts right and don't make up rights that don't exist.

15. Be polite to the doctors/nurses/receptionists, etc. Don't doubt my parentage because I won't see you before the really sick bloke in Resus. A thank you and a compliment can really make a difference to our day and might get you further along than complaining.

16. Don't be racist. Ever. The NHS would collapse if it were not for foreign and non-Caucasian staff. The phrase 'I ain't seeing no Paki doctor' will end up with you 'ain't seeing no doctor'.

17. Don't be homophobic. I am told that 96.7 per cent of

all male A&E nurses are gay (and they are working hard to convert the other 3.3 per cent). *Please note that this is not an accurate figure, just a joke... the true figure is much, much higher.*

18. If you are from a nursing home and confused, please bring a carer who cares about you and knows why the matron has sent you to A&E.

19. If you think we have been nice to you, please write in to say thanks. It really does make our day worthwhile – genuinely.

20. Make jokes with us, but please make them funny.

21. Don't flirt with the nurses or female doctors – that's my job.

22. When you see us at the desk, don't moan loudly that we are sitting having a chat – we are writing notes and getting advice from specialist doctors. We are only occasionally just having a chat.

23. When asked what happened, try to get to the point in under 10 minutes.

24. Similarly, if describing an assault, don't explain in detail why it 'weren't your fault'.

25. Don't ask female doctors 'When am I going to see the doctor please, nurse?'.

26. When I introduce myself as the Registrar don't ever say 'I came here for my chest and not to get married! ha-ha-ha.'

27. If I make a joke – please laugh.

28. Understand I am allowed to yawn at 4 a.m. in the middle of a 12-hour shift so don't say 'Am I keeping you up?'

29. When the speciality team I have referred you to asks you the same questions I did earlier, try and answer with the same answers.

30. If you don't agree with what I am doing let me know ASAP – I am not a policeman, or a prison warden. I can't keep you in hospital against your will. So tell me you are going to self-discharge before I have organised expensive tests and a bed.

31. Have a condition we can treat in less than 4 hours to the point of discharge or to admission. Don't come with complicated problems which might mean time-consuming tests – we can't have you breaking our precious 4-hour rule, now can we?

32. Understand that we have emotions too. We may have just seen a child die, or had to break bad news to a relative. It may be our sixth night in a row, and we might be missing our family. We may be carrying emotional baggage with us which our professional façade does not allow us to expose to the outside world. Have patience with us, be polite and friendly and don't moan too much if you have to wait to be seen.

33. If you follow 1–32, you can (hopefully) expect good quality, timely treatment from A&E staff.

The effects of bloody accounting rules

It's not just me who gets annoyed with how accounting rules forget about patients. I went to a conference last week and heard a story about a patient from a fellow A&E doctor. He was 45 and fed up (the patient not the doctor – she was 33 and fed up) and came in because he didn't know what else to do. He had tingling in his thumb, index and middle finger – its called carpel tunnel syndrome. The irritation was so bad that he was having trouble sleeping. He had had it seen by his GP and had been referred to the local surgeon, who, with a couple of minor cuts to the structures in his wrist, could resolve his problem. However, he hadn't seen the surgeon yet or had the operation. The surgeon had available time, there were some brand spanking new theatres to do the operation in and the day ward had a lot of free space because the local private treatment centre had nicked most of their patients. The actual additional costs for the NHS (sutures, scalpels, bandages, etc.) would have been very minimal – the fixed costs (surgeon, nurses and theatre) had already been met. The problem was that new budget rules mean the PCT pays for each individual operation and his local trust was much overspent. He had had his referral delayed until after April as it would then be in the new financial year. As he had waited less than 18 weeks, the PCT still met its targets. The manager was happy as the cost was delayed for the local PCT until after April, and the government could say that it had fulfilled its targets.

The people who weren't happy were the surgeon and theatre staff, who were bored with twiddling their thumbs, and the

A&E doctor who had to give out strong pain killers at 2 a.m., for a problem that could have been sorted out weeks ago. And let's not forget, most importantly, the patient.

I don't profess to understand the details of accounting and I have limited financial management skills (hence my excessive credit card bills) but surely this is madness. When NHS finances and organisations are not cooperative, but competitive, then middle managers cannot see the wood for the trees. In this case they couldn't see that saving a small amount of money for the PCT would cost the hospital a lot of money, cause resentment in the hospital workers and piss off a patient. Well done, Mr Blair, on producing such a ridiculously managed NHS.

Please come to A&E

You may have noticed that I frequently moan about people who come to A&E unnecessarily. However, today I had a patient that I just couldn't believe didn't want to 'bother us'. He was a 55-year-old builder. Six days previously he had spilt molten hot tarmac on his arm. He didn't want to bother anyone, so he put some cream and a dressing on it. It was still painful, but he still didn't want to be a nuisance so he just took more and more analgesia. It was only when he took off his shirt and a work colleague saw his burn that he was persuaded to come to A&E.

He had a small, full-thickness burn, with surrounding partial thickness burn and damage to his nerves. He must have been in agony. I just don't understand how he could have had such a stiff upper lip or not have died already from infection. We sent him straight to the local burns unit where he will stay in for skin grafts but he could very possibly lose the arm.

I have seen many similar cases of people putting up with problems and not seeing a doctor. The most common are chest pain and acute shortness of breath. If you get either of these, come and see us please, and come now. The same advice applies if you pour molten tarmac over your arms.

We have gone drug crazy

I live in a 'high' town. Not in an altitude sense, but in a drug-taking sense. I saw three interesting patients today, all of whom were in because of drug complications.

The first one came in because he was starting to feel very anxious after taking ecstasy – it was his first night on 'E'. I initially tried to calm him down verbally and explain that it was a consequence of the drug, but that didn't work. He just kept on shouting 'I need a beat'. I tried some diazepam but that didn't seem to work either. 'I need to move,' he cried out.

Being a holistic doctor, I decided to go for another tactic. I asked one of my nursing colleagues to come and join me. I instructed her to be a human beat-box. Bemused but compliant, she started going 'boom, boom, boom, boom' to a typical R&B beat. I then added 'oooooooohhhhhh, ooooohhhhh' as an off-beat addition. The patient nodded and started to move to the impromptu performance. Three minutes later he started to feel better and was now calm and compliant. I gave him some more diazepam. He quickly stopped moving, we stopped our beat-box routine and he fell asleep on the trolley. He was discharged relaxed and happy 5 hours later (or 4 hours as was probably put on the computer.)

I then saw the effects of a cocktail of drugs including ketamine (on an unconscious teenager, with very worried parents). Because of his level of unconsciousness he needed to be intubated and his airway protected so that he didn't choke on his own vomit. He ended up in the ITU for three days at a large cost to you and me as tax payers.

The next patient I saw was a 29-year-old who had given himself chest pains by taking too much cocaine. Cocaine is thought of as a safe, 'trendy' drug. It is not. It is powerfully psychologically addictive and can cause spasm of the coronary arteries. This is what had happened to this patient and he was soon sent to the CCU, where he was the youngest patient by about 40 years. He soon came down from his high, but his cardiac damage is permanent.

It is fascinating working in A&E as you see such weird and wonderful side-effects of drugs. It is also very scary. All three patients had responsible jobs and when at work had others in their care.

Coming home for Christmas

I was really pissed off I was working this Xmas Day. I really wanted it off, so I could spend it with my family. But, unfortunately, people get ill outside 9 – 5 Monday to Friday and so I suppose it is something that you sign up to when you choose this job… until you are a boss and you can get your juniors to do most of the unsocial shifts.

My mild annoyance soon dissipated very quickly, however, with the arrival of the shift's first 'major'. A young lad in his 20s had been involved in a road traffic accident and he was arriving in 10 minutes. (The new term is apparently 'road traffic incident' as the traffic police say the word 'accident' implies that nobody was at fault and it was a random occurrence. This is hardly ever the case.)

As the classic song goes, he had been 'driving home for Christmas'. What isn't in the song was that he was driving home for Christmas very fast, as he was going to be late for his festivities. He had also been out late, enjoying a Christmas Eve piss up. We found out later, that even though it was 10 a.m., he was still over the limit despite finishing his partying 8 hours before.

We got the call from the ambulance team at 10 a.m. He had been travelling at 90 mph. No other car was involved, but he seemed to have flipped his car and it skidded 50 metres upside down. He was the only passenger. Luckily, he had been wearing a seat belt and the air bags had been deployed. I called for the trauma team, which is made up of anaesthetists, surgeons and orthopaedic surgeons who are 'on-call' but during the day are based on the wards and in operating theatres, doing day-to-day work. They come down to A&E when we need their additional help and expertise to manage a trauma. Usually, the trauma is led by an A&E doctor like me, who is in overall charge of the situation while the casualties are in the department. My job is to coordinate everyone, to get a 'wide-angled lens' view of what needs to be done (as opposed to just concentrating on a specific part of the body), to organise definite care and scans and to explain to the patient what is happening.

As soon as the patient came in, I realised that he needed no explanations. His head was bleeding and he was unconscious. After an initial examination, we realised that both his legs were broken. Fortunately, initial examinations showed that his chest and abdomen were not badly damaged.

The main problem was his head. There are two immediate risks in this type of situation. First, that he might vomit and inhale, and then the vomit would clog his lungs and hamper his breathing. Second, if he had a bleed in his brain, then the pressure in his brain would grow and eventually crush the area of the brain responsible for breathing – also not so good.

Both of these are managed by intubating the patient (i.e. putting him to sleep and taking over his breathing). While the anaesthetists were doing this, the orthopaedic surgeons and I tried to stop some of the bleeding from the broken legs. This generally involves pulling the fractured bones back into alignment. There is no great science to it. Just pull it to the angle that looks right. They can be sorted out properly at a later date; he had more pressing issues.

He was intubated and we phoned the radiology consultant to come in to do a full-body scan and then interpret if for us. Amazingly, there was no argument and the radiologist was in the hospital within 10 minutes – grumpy, as usual, but at least he was here.

The CT scan showed a large bleed in the brain, which meant he was probably going to be badly disabled for life – either that or die in the next 48 hours. Which one is worse, I am not sure. Plans were made for transferring him to the local specialist neurosurgical (brain surgery) hospital, so they could operate to drain the blood and relieve the pressure on his brain.

In the meantime, the anaesthetists were giving drugs to reduce the pressure in the brain and prevent further damage. It was my job was to talk to the family.

Even though most of my best medical practice is done with my mouth rather than my stethoscope, and even though I have broken bad news countless times, I was dreading this. I hate it, but someone has got to do it, and I feel that I am as good as any of the other doctors on the team at this job. I took one of the nurses in with me as support, both for me and the family.

As I started to talk to them, I felt the slight depersonalisation that I often get. I found myself looking down on myself speaking to them. It doesn't stop me being compassionate, but it does protect my mental health.

I felt awful. There was I talking them through what had and was going to happen. At the same time I found myself holding the mother's hand as it felt the right thing to do – reassuring and comforting. But at the same time, I also felt that it was like an episode of *EastEnders* – his mum was blaming herself for having a go at him earlier as he might be late for lunch. He had even told her that he would drive like the wind so that he wouldn't be late. Meanwhile, the dad wanted to know if he had been over the limit from last night's festivities. Apparently, he had been with his cousin, who apparently was a 'good-for-nothing little shit', who always made his son drink to excess and who 'was going to pay for this'.

His sister brought some sensibility to the discussion.

'Is he going to… ?' she didn't say the word die, but I knew what she was asking.

'I don't know. We are doing everything we can but he has been seriously injured.'

'Don't let him die,' pleaded his mum.

I didn't know what to do so I just frowned. She gave me a hug and begged me to save him.

'We will do our best,' I said. That was the truth, but I wasn't sure if it was going to be good enough.

It was a shit start to my Christmas but it stopped me moaning about being at work. I looked at the box of the next few patients who were waiting – two chest pains, an asthmatic having an attack, an injured finger, a sore throat and tooth ache. Thank God that these are the normal type of patients we see in A&E. Thankfully, the trauma case is a rarity, otherwise I am not sure that I could handle this job.

It came to home time, and I called my mother-in-law's house to say I was going to be a bit late for Christmas dinner. My wife was a bit miffed, but after I told her what had happened she certainly didn't moan or ask me to speed home.

On the way home, I had a few thoughts. What if he dies? Not just from a 'what a catastrophe for his family' point, but from a professional perspective. If he dies, the family will not blame the medical staff. If he survives, however, we will get the credit and praise. This is very different from most doctors – if a GP misses a diagnosis then they can be vilified. If someone dies in a routine operation, the surgeon will be investigated and their career damaged. But in cases like this we very rarely get blamed as the cause of the injuries are out of everyone's control.

The downside to this is that people very rarely realise that the quality of care affects the outcome – they just blame the initial injury. They believe it was an inevitable outcome from the accident, not one that might have had an alternative ending in a different hospital with different resources and differently trained staff. I am not saying we are responsible for everyone who dies from a trauma. Cases like this involve everyone working their hardest to provide the best possible care. However, we are limited by our resources and the skills and experience of the members of the team, and this can affect the outcome in these types of patients.

What the lack of public awareness of this means is that there is a lack of public pressure to improve the care for emergency patients. There are thousands of cancer charities, but very few that promote 'pre-hospital care' and even fewer campaigning for the improved care of trauma victims. This is despite trauma being the leading cause of death in the young adult population. It has been shown that better care and facilities lead to better outcomes. Greater investment in A&E care would massively alter the outcomes of many of these patients. Of course, in many cases even the best care in the world could not alter some outcomes, but in many, simply improving research funding and resources could save many lives and decrease morbidity. The decreased morbidity would soon save millions in not having to pay sick benefit and having people back at work and paying taxes. Even government accountants should agree with that spending increase.

Other factors lowering the political interest are the heterogeneity of trauma cases: it is very hard to try and get meaningful trauma survival rates for each hospital as opposed to say, cancer mortality rates. This lack of a target means that the government is not as interested in the quality of care. It wants a target to show off to the voters, so for A&E it has produced a 4-hour waiting target, rather than a quality of care one, which ends up distorting priorities. However, politically it makes sense as there are a lot more voters who have had to wait to get their stubbed toe seen to than have been in a near-fatal accident.

The lack of political interest in trauma outcomes also means there is only a tiny amount of public investment into trauma research. Where there is investment in research, it is often heavily restricted into what can and cannot be researched. Politicians are concerned about not doing trials on people without their express consent (which is very hard to get from an unconscious trauma patient), which means that research into how best to care for these people is very difficult to do in this country. There is currently a worldwide research trial into whether a particular drug that stops bleeding would be of benefit in patients such as the one described. But the UK is one of the lowest contributors to the data because of the complexities of taking part in the trial. We didn't enter the patient into the trial purely because the amount of bureaucracy involved would have made it very difficult. He potentially didn't get a beneficial drug and neither will future patients because of difficulties constructed by research committees in this country.

Added to this are the budgetary constraints being instituted across the NHS. Two things that have been cut, and no-one seems to have noticed, will soon affect the care of trauma patients. First, there is a Trauma Audit Research Network which hospitals pay to join. For their money, researchers look at the patient notes, collate data and look at how well they are managing their trauma patients, then recommend how they can improve their care. Some hospitals are saving money by not joining this network and thus are not getting the vital feedback they need.

Second, the study budgets for nurses and doctors are being cut. These study budgets, in the past, have been used to pay for high-quality trauma training – Advanced Trauma Life Support (ATLS) courses. Less funding means fewer staff being able to attend the courses, which means less well trained doctors and nurses looking after you, which means you may have a worse outcome. These cuts have not even entered anyone's political debate but then I suppose we shouldn't complain about the NHS not having enough money. The government needs the money for other vital things such as paying for a war in Iraq and renewing the Trident missile system...

As I thought about this, I got more and more annoyed – why do I mull over things so much after work and why do all my thoughts end up with me becoming angry, ranting and usually getting political? It must really drive my family and friends mad as this is all I think about. So, one of my New Year's resolutions must be to not think about work on my drive home, otherwise I'll send myself mad.

I decided to start my New Year's resolution early. I put on the radio and listened to some inane presenter encouraging me to sing along to 'Rocking around the Christmas Tree' and then 'Mistletoe and Wine'. For the first time ever, I found Cliff Richard relaxing and enjoyable. That is something else I better hide from my friends and family.

ℒ The joys of shift work

One of the lows of workings as an A&E doctor is the effect shift work has on your body clock. I notice a number of problems. First, I just can't wake up easily before going to work and second, my bowels go crazy. Things got bad last night before work.

My wife tried the normal tactic of gently kissing me at first, then nudging me and then pulling off the covers, before resorting to pouring cold water over me – all with no effect. She has learned that she needs to start getting me up quite early as I take a while to rouse. Her latest tactic has been to start a countdown until I have to leave, with increasing levels of threats of violence if I don't get up. Tonight, however, was worse than usual. The routine shouting soon started.

'Nick it is eight-fifteen. Get up' – no response from me

'Nick it is EIGHT-THIRTY. GET UP NOW!!!' Again, no response.

'NICK. GET UP NOW. IT IS EIGHT-FORTY. GET UP NOW!!!' She bellowed up the stairs.

It was only when my mobile went off and I saw a text message from my next door neighbour that I realised that I need to get in to a better routine before work. It read 'Nick. Apparently it is 8.40. I think you need get up and go to work!' Oh, the joys of shift work and terraced housing.

The other main problem is what shift work does to your bowels at night. I have nicknamed it SWAC (shift worker's anal conditions) as a main term and I suffer from two subtypes – nocturnal SACS (sweaty arse-crack syndrome) and nocturnal

CATED (constipation and then excessive diarrhoea). Luckily, it all goes back to normal once I am on day shifts. I am so looking forward to the coming stretch of six weeks of days before my wife loses her voice and my arse becomes an issue again.

Careful with your notes and coffee room chats

In the last couple of months, I have listened to two of the most amusing talks. One by the hospital solicitors and one by the Medical Protection Society – a doctor's legal advice service. Both were about how to write in notes and not get sued. Two main bits of advice were given. First, write what you have done. If it is not in the notes, then it hasn't happened. Second, be careful about what is written. Do not use acronyms – especially TLAs – three letter acronyms – it leads to confusion. Do not insult people (they can now get hold of your notes) and don't use insulting acronyms (it is the worst of both worlds).

With this on board, and knowing that I was a new breed of doctor who was too scared of being struck off to do any of this (and also someone who believes patients should automatically get a copy of their attendance letter from A&E), all I could do was sit back and enjoy what some others had written in the past... and you thought that all doctors were angelic creatures. *(Please note that although I think that the following comments may be potentially amusing, they are insulting and should never be used.)*

Diagnosis

NFB – normal for Birmingham.

FLK syndrome – funny-looking kid

FLP with a FLK – funny-looking parent with a funny-looking kid (the condition is often hereditary).

FLKBOFB – funny-looking kid, but OK for Birmingham.

FLKNLP – funny-looking kid, normal-looking parents (the kid's condition has not been inherited).

GOMER – get out of my emergency room. Used for old patient who is ill and you need to admit them to a ward before they become really ill and become your problem.

RIP – rest in peace. Nothing rude about that, except beneath the notes certifying the death, a doctor had drawn a grave stone with some flowers around it and then written RIP on the gravestone.

TFTB – too fat to breathe.

WNL (as in 'observations were all WNL') – within normal limits/we never looked.

ECG (heart tracing), **NAD** – no abnormalities detected/not actually done.

COPD – chronic obstructive respiratory disorder/chronic old person disorder.

PEP – pharmacologically enhanced personality (pissed or stoned).

CRAFT – can't remember a f**king thing.

NPS – new parent syndrome. Parent anxious. Child well.

Oligoneuronal – not many brain cells (similarly used is pneumocranial – air head, literally air in the head).

LPT – low pain threshold.

PFO/DFO – pissed fell over/drunk fell over.

ASS – arrest avoidance syndrome. Similar to PAS (prison avoidance syndrome) and PDSD (pre-detention stress disorder).

PTSD – post truncheon stress disorder. Similar to above but also involves trying to make up symptoms or blame previous injuries on the police.

TATT – tired all the time.

TTT ratio – teeth to tattoo ratio. A low ratio implies a difficult upbringing with all the cosmetic effects that has on people.

ONF – overall nick factor.

As I said earlier, these terms are rightly consigned to the history books. I always write notes knowing that patients can read them and I don't want to cause upset. However, one place where they are still used is A&E coffee rooms. There are also a lot of slang terms used in these rooms, and since I am trying to show what it is like to work in A&E, understanding some of these terms is quite important.

Can't Decide Unit – other name for Clinical Decision Unit. The bit of A&E where we put all the patients in who have been there for more than 4 hours so they don't break the 4-hour target.

Meet, treat and street nurses – triage nurses who can now put on a sticky plaster and then say goodbye.

Code blue – a really non-urgent ambulance that should never have been called.

Smurf positive – blue colour of patient owing to hypoxia/ lack of oxygen.

Simpson positive – a patient with jaundice.

Homer Simpson positive – a gay patient with jaundice.

Rooney fracture – fracture of the fourth metatarsal.

Beckham fracture – fracture of the fifth metatarsal.

An Owen knee – knee pointing in the wrong direction (as per Michael Owen in the 2006 World Cup).

Ear ring sign – the larger the hooped earring, the more likely she is to have pelvic inflammatory disease as opposed to appendicitis. Similar to the toe ring and ankle bracelet sign.

Granny dumped – happens on Christmas Eve, when family want to go on holiday. Speaks for itself.

Gomergram – GOMER who you do a battery of tests on if you have no idea what is going on (ECG, chest X-ray, blood tests and in America a CT scan).

Buff – make the patient easier to refer to another team (i.e. moderate chest pain, gets exaggerated to excruciating chest pain).

Turf – send to another team so it is not our problem.

Fluttering eye syndrome – a patient who fakes unconsciousness, but we know they are making it up as they flutter their eyelids when you stroke them.

O sign – old person dying with their mouth open.

Q sign – old person dying with their mouth open and tongue out.

Dotted Q sign – old person dying with their mouth open and tongue out and fly on the tongue.

Chav – English equivalent of trailer trash. Not really sure what it stands for. A policeman friend of mine claims that it means 'Council Housing and Violent'.

Chavet – female chav.

Chavlett – young chav.

Ash cash – money for signing cremation forms. Personally, I think that the amount of money people pay for us to sign a form, so that they can cremate their relatives, is disgusting. However, I am hypocritical and happily spend the money. In quite a sick way lots of junior doctors buy rounds and then toast the person whose family has just paid for the drinks.

Ash machine – a doctor's cash machine.

A part 2 slimer – a doctor who makes friends with the morticians, purely so they can get to fill in parts of the cremation forms and make lots of money.

Bash cash – money the police give us for describing the beating that we treated in A&E.

To an outsider, these may seem sick and cruel words, but they are used away from patients and are part of the black humour that keeps A&E staff sane. So, be wary of going into a staff room in any hospital and, please note, my describing these terms does not mean that in any way do I approve of them.

An embarrassed husband

Working in A&E you always get to see a few patients with rectal foreign bodies – things placed where they shouldn't be. It's an occupational hazard of anal play, but it's not my cup of tea. However, it really doesn't bother me at all if that's how you like to get your kicks. I don't get embarrassed by it (much) and I often feel genuinely sorry for the patients. They are very embarrassed and doctors and nurses can only make it worse by asking too many questions or taking a moralistic view.

There a few cases that spring to mind. However, there is only one that is truly memorable, but mostly for the reaction of a fellow doctor to the patient. The gentleman in question came in with a 'personal problem', and he had asked to be seen somewhere private. I asked what had happened. He started to lie – it was obvious.

'I was lying on the couch and fell asleep. I had taken my trousers off because I spilt wine on them. Then my phone went. I went to pick it up off the sofa and I slipped and it sort of... '

'Is there a phone up your rectum sir?' I asked. He nodded nervously. 'Don't worry. It doesn't bother me. I am only here to help you.' I didn't ask what make, or if it was on vibrate mode.I X-rayed his abdomen and there it was – from the look of it probably a Nokia 6250i or something similar. I just hoped that it wouldn't ring. There was no way that it would come out without a general anaesthetic and the skills of a good surgeon. Some foreign bodies even need a cut to be made in the abdomen so that they can be pushed out from the inside so to speak. I explained all this to him.

'But you must get it out now; my wife can't know... she doesn't know about that side of me and I don't want to lose my kids.' He started to panic.

I explained that there was no alternative. Leaving it there was a definite no-no as it might perforate the bowel and cause septicaemia and death.

He continued to panic. He explained to me that his wife was a medical secretary at a local GP practice and would have access to any notes sent to his GP about the episode. I assured him that no notes would be made available to his wife and that we wouldn't tell her anything. However, that didn't satisfy him.

'I can't have the operation or my marriage is over. I am leaving,' he whispered. I tried to stop him leave and then offered him a solution.

'You could lie. We can't lie for you, but you could say you have an anal fissure that has started to bleed and they need to do an examination under anaesthetic.'

He seemed a little calmer now. I phoned the surgical team on call and explained to them what had happened and his embarrassing predicament. I explained to them the explanation I had given him to offer to his wife, so that they would know what he was going to say so they didn't put their foot in it. The response I got shocked me.

'You can lie if you want, but it's his sin and his problem. I am not taking part in your deceit.'

I didn't see the patient after that. I hope the surgeon was a little bit more understanding of his predicament face to face, otherwise, if it ever happened again, then the patient would be too embarrassed to come back to A&E and could end up with the complications of foreign bodies where they shouldn't be – septicaemia and death. It is not our job to moralise but we often do and sometimes you can't help it. However, part of the job is hiding your own views from the patients.

℞ The human effect of reconfiguration and lack of beds

Just in case you thought that the NHS emergency care reconfiguration was a utopia of improved health, I want to remind you of the reality.

A 19-year-old patient had been involved in a massive car accident. He needed his breathing taken over for him and for that he needed to go to ICU. The only problem was that there were no ICU beds available. This was not a new problem but had been exacerbated by an increase in serious cases coming to our hospital as the other local A&E had, in all but name, been closed. However, the genius planners had not considered the fact that the only hospital in the region with a fully functioning A&E would now have a busier ICU. Consequently, there had been not enough increase in funding and not enough new beds were funded for all the extra patients.

The problem of a lack of ICU beds existed before the reconfiguration, but now in my hospital it is a lot worse. In this case the patient, instead of going to ICU, stayed in A&E till they could 'create' a bed. This involved waiting for a ward patient to die, a high-dependency patient going into their bed, a patient from ICU going to the high-dependency unit (HDU) ward and then quickly cleaning the spare ICU bed.

This meant that an anaesthetist had to stay with the patient for 6 hours until they were on ICU. This in turn meant that the appendicitis case that I referred 4 hours ago, and the patient who needed a 'ERPC' – removal of an embryo after a miscarriage – who both were due for an operation that night, were delayed. Those patients were unduly put at psychological, if not a serious medical, risk. Not knowing this, they did not make a fuss.

Another patient who suffered was a gentleman needing his oesophagus removed for cancer. His surgery was booked for the next day. However, it is a very large operation and he would need an ICU bed post-op. As there now were none, the operation was postponed. All these patients were told it was an exceptionally busy night, no-one could have predicted it, etc., etc. They were not told that the root cause was poor managerial planning.

So, the inpatients had their length of stay increased and their cost to the NHS rose. The cancer patient had another few days' wait for the operation and the surgeon and his team sat frustrated that they couldn't operate.

Reconfigurations without proper planning have made our hospital ICU run at close to 100 per cent bed occupancy. What managers must realise is that this leads to decreased efficiency and care. It is not just ICUs running at close to 100 per cent occupancy, but the whole hospital. Surely the managers have got to realise that the point about emergency care is that it is unpredictable and you need to have spare capacity to cope with minor surges in need. Even the Department of Health in 2002 said that the optimum bed occupancy rate is 82 per cent. However, week-in, week-out we go above this and patients do suffer. That's why you need clinical advisors when a hospital needs a 'hit squad' to come and improve things, not some city kids in suits, who are called management consultants, charge a grand a day and know bugger-all about patient care.

While I am on the case about managers, it is important to realise that there are a massive number of excellent ones working in the NHS. But they have to implement politicians' plans and with limited resources and skewed targets. I need to remember that when I get frustrated with them.

Unexpected laughter

Today, I had a tragedy turn into a comedic episode. I had to certify a patient's death and the family ended up in fits of giggles. It was a very odd experience and just shows that people cope with grief in different ways. The patient, who eventually died, came in from the ambulance in 'cardiac arrest'. She had no heartbeat and the ambulance personnel were doing chest compressions.

During the cardiac arrest, I was supervising one of the junior doctors on how to 'run' a cardiac arrest – she was doing very well. However, cardiac arrests are not like you see them on TV. Only rarely are they successful – this is partly because we have all forgotten the importance of actually compressing the chest properly when the heart stops, as opposed to giving fancy drugs – for which there is little evidence that they make any difference. Patients also rarely wake up and say thank you and walk out. They go to ICU and three days later they may or may not wake up with some brain damage. After 15 minutes we realised that this case was 'futile'. We couldn't save her. My junior colleague quite rightly asked if we all agreed to stop her chest compressions. Everyone nodded.

She was placed into the 'quiet room' ready to transfer to the 7th floor (we have only six floors and it is a euphemism for the mortuary). The family was by her side – her daughter and three grandchildren. Before she could be moved to the chapel of rest, she had to be formally certified. This was the first 'cardiac arrest' my junior colleague had been in charge of. I therefore offered to certify on her behalf while she composed herself.

I had already met the family and explained what had happened to their mother, and so had no problems speaking to them again. I explained what I needed to do, and asked if they wished to stay. They did. I then asked if they had any questions. They did. The youngest of the grandchildren spoke.

'Did you used to live in Stanford Drive?'

'Why?' I asked.

'A few years ago?' he asked.

I nodded and again asked why.

'See, I told you all,' he said to his family. Looking back at me, he continued, 'Did you used to have a dodgy "kung fu fighting" dressing gown?' he asked.

'Yes, when I was a student. As soon as I went out with my wife, she chucked out all my clothes and I became well dressed. Why?' I really wasn't expecting this type of questioning and was becoming a bit perturbed. I think my facial expression was showing that now.

'And did you used to have your milk delivered?' he continued.

In a rather shocked way, not expecting my retail preferences to being the main points discussed in this meeting, I nodded. He seemed to take glee from this and said to his family once again. 'Told you so!'

He turned to me.

'I used to be your milkman mate... Tony. Do you remember?'

I smiled and everyone burst into laughter. Had he more to say?

'Word of advice mate. Wear boxers with that dressing gown. It was a bit too see-through if you know what I mean.'

He burst out in tears of laughter and I couldn't stop myself smiling and nervously joined in with the laughing. All the time his grandma lay dead between us. It was a very surreal experience and his mother could obviously tell my unease.

'Don't worry, love. She liked a good joke and tease. It's a tribute to her that we can still laugh about things.'

As I walked out of the room still laughing my junior colleague walked past.

'Why are you laughing?' she asked.

'I've just certified the death of our last patient and I haven't been so amused for days.'

I needed to do some explaining before I was thought of as the most insensitive doctor ever to have existed...

Repeat attenders

Some patients I love treating – others I don't. I have just finished a set of seven nights and seen the same bloke five times. Each time he has come in drunk, with nothing wrong. Each night he makes up a symptom. He is homeless and there is nothing wrong with him except that when it is raining he wants a bed for the night. He can't get a hostel because he won't stop drinking. It is a very difficult situation and very hard to discharge people into the cold outside. We can't give in to his demands because otherwise it would set a precedent and we wouldn't have the beds to look after people who genuinely needed them for medical reasons. His problems need to be sorted out by society.

On the fourth night it was very cold and raining and he refused to leave. He started getting loud and swearing and began upsetting the children in the department. We had to get security to escort him off the premises. As soon as he left he called an ambulance from the nearest phone box and complained of suicidal tendencies and came back. Eventually, we had to call the police. I explained to him that I couldn't let him stay for the night. He asked the police if they could take him for the night. They shook their heads and tried to escort him off the premises again.

'You can only get a bed if you get nicked mate,' they informed him, much to our cost. He then kicked the window of our A&E and smashed it. They nicked him and he got what he wanted. What a sad reflection on society.

While I don't blame him for wanting somewhere warm for the night, it was very frustrating for all concerned.

This job is hard

As an A&E doctor, you sometimes have to develop a barrier where you don't let emotion get to you. It is important, because only by being rational can you deliver good quality care. But sometimes little things get to you and however hardened you are your emotions can buckle. This morning I buckled.

It was 7 a.m. Only 2 hours before home time. A fry-up and a pint of beer with the 9.30 a.m. regulars at my local

Wetherspoon's (the shift workers and enthusiastic drinkers) beckoned. But then the red phone went off: 14-year-old girl, overdose, unconscious.

We called down the anaesthetic team, in case we had to take over the care of her breathing, and also called the paediatricians. She came in and I went into autopilot. You learn a set routine. Check her airway, give oxygen and check her breathing, check her pulse rate and blood pressure and then give fluids. Basically, stabilise the patient and then think. She was soon stabilised and not in any immediate danger. I soon realised that the mum was standing near us. Out of autopilot, I went to comfort her and explain what had happened.

'Nick', the senior sister called out. 'Her blood pressure has fallen.' Some of then drugs she had taken had caused that. Back onto autopilot. No emotions. More venous access obtained and another drip put up.

Soon her condition had turned from serious to stable and I was able to get some history about what had happened from her mum. I asked her if she knew why her daughter had taken the drugs. She cried and handed me a suicide note as she muttered about bullying.

The letter was heartbreaking; it described the feelings of hopelessness that she felt and how she saw no other option to stop the endless cycle of bullying and self loathing. It was the saddest thing I have ever read. She apologised to her parents and asked them to carry on looking after her guinea pig.

I read it and the experience of reading her thoughts made me shudder and think. It put my concerns into perspective. I couldn't stop thinking of her parents. How will they cope if she dies? Then I had a selfish thought. Why do I put myself through this? Am I strong enough to cope with experiences like this? I should be in bed by now, cuddling my own child and telling them how much I love them. It is always hard in situations like this, not to let them affect you personally, but this is often very hard to do. So why do I put myself through this stuff? The answer is simple. Because of all the work we all did, her mum got a chance to tell her she loves her too. I couldn't swap this job for another even if it costs me lots in Kleenex tissues – which you can't even claim for against tax.

P.S. She was transferred to the regional centre of paediatric intensive care and made a good recovery.

Another sad case

I saw an 82-year-old gentleman today. His wife had died earlier that month. He was brought in after he was spotted at a local beauty spot with a hose going into his car from his exhaust. The fire brigade broke into the car and the ambulance brought him in.

This was a genuine attempted suicide case. He told me that he had lived for his wife. He had no children and few friends. All he wanted to do was join her in the 'afterlife'. He couldn't cope with the loneliness. He told me that his decision was a logical one, made by a man who had full faculties of mind. He told me that as soon as I had discharged him, he would try and kill himself again. He told me that that was the right thing for him to do, so that he could join her in heaven. He was lonely and missing her.

I sympathised greatly, but still asked the psychiatrist to see him, knowing that they would admit him to a psychiatric hospital. I have no idea if I did the right thing but I was sure that if he left then he would kill himself. I just didn't know if that was the best thing for him. In all honesty, I referred him to the psychiatrist because I had to. I didn't want to feel the guilt if he did kill himself and I didn't want to face a coroner's court case where I admitted discharging someone who had an acute depressive episode.

The importance of banter at work

The department got a complaint letter today. It said that the doctors writing their notes seemed to be chatting too much with the nurses and there was too much 'fun' going on. We then all got told by our bosses to 'cut out the banter'.

Doctors and nurses do need to be careful about how we act in areas where the public can see us. But we need to be careful not to lose the camaraderie that a bit of banter can bring about. It helps keep up morale and can therefore improve patient care. Please just remember that when you see doctors and nurses having a chat (we may even be discussing important clinical information).

One of the best things about working nights is that there is more opportunity for banter – or team building as I like to call it. There are no bosses, fewer patients and the ones who are there are usually pissed as a fart. In some A&Es doctors and nurses have been known to play 'games' with the patients – although this is only done if they are drunk and never if anyone is distressed, ill or sober enough to know what they are doing.

There is the game of seeing how many song titles from various albums you can get into one short consultation. There is the very similar and somewhat more amusing game of trying to get a bizarre but relevant fact into a consultation. These games are only possible because of the fact that all A&E consultations occur behind curtains – which are not soundproof, and so an independent adjudicator can mark you. Again, just because I am talking about these things doesn't necessarily mean that I approve.

Only when it gets quiet and the A&E department is left empty can the fun really begin. Most times an empty A&E leads to the staff trying to get a bit of rest or people surfing the net. However, if you are on duty with a 'good bunch' of doctors and nurses, then an empty A&E can lead to some great fun and games. Unfortunately, anything you might have thought about such as 'the key game' or 'spin the bottle' is purely for the imaginary letter pages of *Fiesta* or *Escort*: the stock cupboard is usually full of stock and the sluice is probably the least erotic place I can imagine. The A&E games can be much more fun: crutch races, wheelchair races, gloves turned into balloons and then volley ball matches. There are also the practical, slightly macabre, practical jokes to play on the more junior staff. Then there is the routine of drenching with water anyone that has managed to nod off to sleep. These types of things help us cope with the stresses of A&E work at night and also keep us alert in case an emergency comes in.

The best part of nights nowadays is that you can actually have a drink after a night at work. One of the best 'nights' out

I have had recently was when all of us had just finished our last night (of a run of seven) and went out 'morning' drinking. After a change of clothes, we went for a fry-up, and then hit the pub at 9 a.m.; eight of us drinking and playing silly pub games till lunchtime. We were then ready for a club and a kebab, but as it was only noon we went home to our beds instead. Sadly, it is not a truly 24-hour city that I reside in.

The wonders of the Internet

Have you ever been to A&E and for some bizarre reason the doctor has said 'I'll just be a minute' then disappears for 20 minutes? That used to be because the doctor was off to ask someone's advice or look something up in a book. While we know many things, often we get stumped.

Now we have the Internet and it has revolutionised things. We can look up symptoms or rare conditions or sometimes just refresh our memories of long-forgotten diseases last heard about in medical school. Often we say 'I'll just be a minute' to go and look up the latest treatment guidelines on the 'net'. One of my favourite (A&E) sites is called Best-Bets, which basically goes through the evidence for what is the best treatment for various conditions. It is a fantastic site and helps enormously; it is one I use very often.

That is until this afternoon, when I 'logged' on to the net with my password and typed in the site details. All I got was a screen saying, 'You have tried to access an inappropriate site. Your manager will be informed. You are reminded that breaches of the computer use code may result in disciplinary dealings.' What an idiot of a computer person; not letting a vital site be used because it has the word 'bets' in it. I am very much looking forward to my disciplinary meeting. Meanwhile, I had to phone up a friend at another hospital to look up what exactly to do on my behalf. Thankfully, my friend is an ophthalmologist and has plenty of free time to help me out when he is at work.

Just a little small moan

Today a son brought his mother into A&E. She had bled from a varicose vein. This was cleaned and bandaged up, but I wanted to a do a blood test on her before we let her go to check that she was OK. I asked him if he could stay for a couple of hours till the blood results were back. He said he couldn't afford to. I enquired why. He showed me the parking prices. I soon realised... the charges are horrendous. It is a tax on being ill or visiting ill relatives. They justify the prices by saying that they are used to pay for NHS services. But isn't that what our taxes are for?

The joys of A&E

Most people, even ones you really don't like, have some redeeming features: someone I met today most people would describe as having not one. They might go on to describe him as the type of person you could only wish to become better strangers with. However, at work I can't jump to those conclusions and am obliged (quite rightly) to treat him in a non-judgmental way and provide appropriate care regardless of the way he treats me or the NHS. Being non-judgmental is sometimes the hardest – but an essential – part of the job.

The person in question is a man in his 30s and is very well known to the police. Every time he gets arrested, he says his chest hurts and so he gets sent to hospital to stop him having to go to the cells (he has done this over 10 times now, at vast expense to the NHS/police/me and you as taxpayers). This time he got arrested for something vaguely serious. So instead of just saying his chest hurt, he said his chest and stomach hurt. He was initially triaged by an Asian nurse and he responded that he would prefer to be seen by a Caucasian member of staff (he put it in a slightly less polite way).

As the senior doctor, I was asked to see him. None of his symptoms fitted any pathology known to me. Despite his belief that he was going to 'die in the next hour' I felt there were few grounds for concern. When I started to examine him, he started screaming out in pain. All his observations were normal. However, everywhere I touched him was 'f**king agony'; again, not fitting any known pathology. I tried to distract him, and when I did, he became pain free. The best way to do this, I find, is to listen to their abdomen/chest with your stethoscope and press down quite hard. They don't realise that you are trying to elicit pain, so stop acting. I assured him that he didn't need any blood tests and that he could go back with the police. I don't think he agreed with my provisional management plan.

'I am telling you I need some f**king blood tests to prove I'm going to die,' he said.

Now, I know that these are the days of patient choice, but I declined to take his advice and act upon his choice of management plan. I advised him of this. Unfortunately, in this litigious and complaint-led society many doctors sometimes succumb to doing unnecessary blood tests due to patient pressure, and just in case there is a problem, as opposed to trusting their clinical skills. I am one of those doctors. However, in this case I was as sure as sure can be that there was nothing wrong.

'I need some tests, or I'll die. Then you'll be sorry. Do you want to come to my funeral?' he enquired. I advised him that I try to avoid my patients' funerals (it doesn't fill me or the mourners with great confidence). I again reiterated my management plan, which also involved his apologising to the nurse that he had sworn at and then kindly leaving.

'You can go now, sir,' I advised him, content that my management had been appropriate.

'I need morphine now, you c***,' he explained to me.

I explained that there was a seven-year-old in the department and she did not need her vocabulary expanding. I also advised him why paracetamol would be a preferable analgesic to morphine, considering his objective pain-level and both drugs' side-effect profiles. He then started becoming very aggressive and swearing and putting other patients at risk.

At this point I asked the police to take him away. However, he collapsed and started to fit, arms and legs shaking rigorously, but still flinching when I brushed against his eyelashes. It was really bad acting. I got down to him on the floor and whispered, 'Stop it. I know what you are playing at.'

He continued pretending to fit.

I tried to respond to the humanitarian part of his personality. 'Look mate, there are some really sick people here. I need to go and check on the man in cubicle four with a heart attack and there is a seven-year-old girl in cubicle fifteen who now knows a lot more swear words and has a dislocated finger. I need to fix it for her.' Still no response. I started to get annoyed. Real patients were here and he was wasting my time.

'Please stop, sir. Stop being selfish.' (I may not have used those exact words – my memory fails me). He continued and so I decided to go into true bullshit mode.

'Sister,' I called out. 'I think he really is fitting. Quick, come. Can you get the largest catheter possible? We haven't got time for local anaesthetic; we need to know his urine function now. Quick, sister, quick!'

All of a sudden he started to wake up and stop fitting. Considering he had been 'fitting' for 5 minutes, he made a very quick recovery.

'I don't know what happened there,' he said, 'and my pain's gone completely. Can I go now please?'

'Yes. I think it was a severe case of AAS, which has resolved. Take care. Goodbye, sir. Always a pleasure, never a chore.' (AAS – arrest avoidance syndrome)

As an aside, I know the police sometimes come in for a lot of flak. But I want to say that all the police I have ever worked with in A&E have been fantastic. How they keep happy and don't show their anger that often when dealing with people like him, I will never know.

Smoking yourself to death

It is not easy giving up smoking. However, it is a lot easier than being told you are going to die of lung cancer.

A gentleman came to A&E after his wife had forced him to. He had had weeks of problems before succumbing to her pressure.

'So what's up?' I enquired.

The typical hesitant-male-being-encouraged-to-talk-by-his-wife conversation ensued. Eventually I found out what had been bothering him – and it wasn't just his wife's nagging.

'I have been losing weight and coughing a lot. But I had to come today because I have coughed up a lot of blood the last two days.' He didn't make direct eye contact, but looked at me as if he was feeling guilty.

I took some more information and asked if I could examine him. The first things that I noticed were his tar-stained hands from years of smoking (he thought that because the cigarettes were low tar, they weren't that dangerous – he believed a myth not denied by the smoking companies). The next thing I noticed was indeed the amount of weight he had lost. His collar was at least two sizes too large and his trousers were falling off him. I examined his chest and while I was doing that, another coughing stint started. I looked at what he was coughing and it was bright red... and there was a lot of it – at least an eggcup-full of bright-red blood. The sight of this made me feel sick.

I stopped my examination to get a line into his veins in case he needed an urgent blood transfusion. I then went back to examining him. Listening to the base of his lungs, I heard odd noises, which just didn't seem right. I asked him to say '99', but only because that is what patients expect us to say – all the information I was going to need, I was going to get from a chest X-ray. (Also, I am not as clever as the respiratory doctors who actually listen back when you whisper 99.) I then moved on to his abdomen. I laid him down flat and started feeling his abdomen. I felt his liver. It was hard and craggy. I felt sick. He probably had a metastatic lung cancer (i.e. a cancer that had spread and that he was going to die from). He must have noted my unconscious facial expression.

'What is it, Doc? What is going on?'

Shit, I need to think of something to say and quickly. 'Erm... well... we need... ' Where had my bullshit ability gone? Where was it when I needed it? Shit! Then a great idea came to me. I put my stethoscope on his chest again. 'Can you say ninety-nine, please?' He did as requested and I had some breathing space. I repeated the request a few more times, pretended to listen, and I collected my thoughts.

'I am not sure what's going on,' I lied. 'I need to do some tests on you. I need to do an X-ray of your chest and some blood tests. When we get those results, I'll have more of an idea.'

'Have I got cancer, sir?' he asked.

I was honest this time. 'I don't know. I suspect you may, but I can't really say much until I have got some test results back.' He seemed satisfied with that response, and then from nowhere I said, 'I hope not though'. Where that came from, or why, I had no idea. What a stupid thing to say. I meant it though; he was a genuinely nice bloke. He was polite, unassuming and obviously doted on his family.

113

'Me too,' his wife responded.

I sent off a battery of blood tests and sent him for his chest X-ray. I looked at the X-ray when it came back. There was a large mass in the lower part of his left lung. His blood tests came back. He was anaemic from coughing up blood. I then looked at his liver test. The counts were very deranged. Finally, his calcium level was very high – probably from the cancer spreading to the bones. You didn't need to be that skilled to come to the obvious diagnosis (you rarely do in medicine). My suspicions were right. All the evidence was pointing to lung cancer. However, you do need to be skilled at how you tell someone they have cancer. That is something that comes from your personality and is hard to teach. It is also something I rarely do in A&E as a diagnosis of cancer is rarely this obvious. I went into the cubicle where he was and asked him if he wanted to go somewhere more private. He declined my offer, but knew what my opening gambit meant.

'I've got it, ain't I? I've got cancer. Tell me. I need to know. Tell me.'

'The tests so far show you may have a lesion on your chest. You also have some blood tests which show that the liver may be damaged. Although I can't confirm you have lung cancer, I think that you might have it. We need to do some more tests.'

His wife was silent. He strangely seemed relieved.

'At least I know what is going on. What happens now?' He said it in a matter of fact way. I felt that he already knew his diagnosis and I had only confirmed his suspicions. It was odd.

'I have to refer you to the medical team who will take over your care from now on. They will organise various special

114

tests where they try and get some of the tissue and send it to the pathologists to confirm if it is a cancer and what type. They will also do scans to see if it has spread anywhere else. Until those other tests come back, I can't say any more.'

I also explained that as the A&E doctor I would not be involved in their care anymore and that any future questions would best be discussed with the specialist team.

As I spoke, I soon realised that he was listening but his wife was not taking it in. They both spoke at the same time.

'How long have I got?' he said.

'He won't die, will he?' she said.

I was honest. I told them that I didn't know what was going to happen. She started to cry and he told her off for crying.

'I need to tell the kids... what do I say?'

If I had thought telling him he had lung cancer was hard, him telling his kids would be a lot harder than what I just faced. I left the cubicle and made them a cup of tea.

Ironically, it is at times like this when I wish I smoked and had an excuse to go outside for 10 minutes to collect my thoughts. Luckily, I don't. One coughing fit when I was 14 put me off for ever.

The next patient I saw was a 60-year-old smoker who had just had a stroke...

Patient choice or patient confusion?

In the past if you were ill, you would go to your GP. If you were very ill, you would go to A&E. Now you have many other options: NHS Direct, your pharmacist, out-of-hours

GPs, acute care centres, walk-in centres, urgent care centres, walk-in GPs, minor injuries units, major trauma centres, private treatment centres and private diagnostic and treatment centres (which is in essence what a hospital is). All of these are designed to give you, the patient, greater choice.

Did you want all this choice, or would you choose to have a functioning, open, good-quality local district general hospital and a GP that you can see when you need to? I know what I would go for.

Putting yourself at risk

There isn't much risk working in A&E compared with other jobs such as the police, fire brigade or army. However, one of the risks you do have is catching diseases from patients.

At 4 a.m. in came a 32-year-old male. He was a heroin user and had cut his arm on a bottle. He needed suturing. I was doing this when I got a 'nick' through my glove and into my hand. It was nobody's fault – a pure accident. I went through the procedure of washing my hand very thoroughly. My colleague then asked him if he would consent to an HIV (human immunodeficiency virus) and hepatitis test. He said he was 'clean' and refused another test. I couldn't force him to have one and so I was in the lurch not knowing what his HIV status was and therefore what my risk was. I discussed it at length with the specialists and was told that the risk of catching HIV were minuscule.

However, it is hard to rationalise your own risk. It is much easier telling other people than telling yourself. I refused their advice and went on post-exposure prophylaxis (anti-HIV drugs) just in case. I felt sick every time I had a tablet. I also had to wait six long, sex-free weeks until I found out that I did not have HIV. That was a real low of working in A&E – especially the sex-free bit.

I know I have mentioned it before, but shouldn't NHS workers have rights as well? Shouldn't we have the right to do blood tests on high-risk patients when we have sustained an injury helping them? If they don't want the results and don't want anything doing then that is their decision, but to not let health-care workers know the risks they are facing is a bit unfair.

The anger of chess

Sometimes I find myself in some truly bizarre conversations with patients, but this is often one of the funniest bits of working in A&E. Last night the police bought in two rather large, scary-looking, biker types who had gotten into a fight at the local pub.

'So what happened?' I asked in a slightly disinterested, my department is very busy, could you not have kissed and made up and not kicked the shit out of each other? type of way.

'He cheated!' my patient said, getting fired up again and pointing to the man opposite handcuffed by two large coppers.

'Right… but what actually happened?' I repeated.

'I moved my king to D4. He thought I had cheated.'

Slightly bemused, I tried to be not too surprised that not

only had he heard of chess but that he was so passionate about it he that he had lost two teeth in its honour.

I went on. 'OK. But how did you get your cut? Was it from a punch, a glass? What happened?'

'Well, he moved his queen illegally. He jumped a pawn and anyone should know you just can't have that.'

'And... ?' I enquired.

'So that's cheating. I retaliated by moving my pawn across.'

It didn't get any better. Eventually, he admitted that he had gotten so drunk that he couldn't remember what happened but that the fight was definitely over chess. It is stories like this that provide the much-needed, light-hearted relief to stressful days at work.

Training to be a consultant

Many registrars are like me, on a training scheme to become a consultant. It involves two mains bits of education. First, there are training days. These are days of lectures where you are taught how things should be done (the gold standard) as opposed to how things are done in reality. They are also a good chance to meet up with friends and be reassured that you are not the only one a bit pissed off at the moment. However, the vast majority of training is done on the shop floor in an apprentice type of way. The quality of this can vary somewhat, but it sometimes opens your eyes to how the experience of consultants really shows when there are real emergencies. It makes you appreciate them and realise that your skills are in need of improvement.

This weekend I experienced a two-day course of intensive medical education. It was powerfully lectured. They were wide-ranging topics and, best of all, the course was free and included all food and accommodation. Yes, I went home to my mum, who not only knows nothing about medicine but even failed her first-aid at work course. However, she still thinks she knows more than me about health and tries to give me her advice.

I had a nose bleed – according to her you must pinch near the forehead and then go to A&E. I had years of nosebleeds that didn't stop before I learned to pinch the soft bit of the nose for 5 minutes and wait until it stops instead. Then my cousin came to see me as he had hurt himself playing football. I advised paracetamol and ibuprofen, but no, apparently my mother knows better. Pain killers hide the true injury and you always need an X-ray. The other incident was my dad complaining about his bad back. I advised losing some weight and taking pain killers. But again I was wrong. There is apparently a fantastic herbal remedy, for only £69.99 from gulliblemiddleagedhousewife.com.

Mum, thank you for putting me through medical school but please let me be the household advisor on medical matters and you can stick to your specialist subject: knowing when I do or do not need a coat to go out in.

The last straw

It is not just me who gets annoyed about events at work. A friend of mine who works in another region told me about an event at work. He had been seeing a really sick 24-year-old asthmatic. My friend started giving him nebulisers and various drug infusions. However, he soon realised that the patient would need his breathing taken over by an anaesthetist otherwise he would die. He 'fast bleeped' the anaesthetist and medical team to come down. They arrived shortly after. Between them, they stabilised the patient and while the anaesthetist was transferring the patient to ICU, he was letting the distraught family know what was going on. One week later the patient was discharged. I have no doubt that my friend saved this man's life. He then went back to the main section of A&E, to sort out the wait that had ensued while he had been busy. He did not expect any praise for what had happened, but didn't expect the criticism he got from his seniors and from management about the number of '4-hour breaches' that ensued on his shift. No wonder he is planning on leaving A&E medicine and becoming a GP – I think this was the last straw. At least when he is a GP, he might feel valued.

Missed fractures

Part of a consultant's job is to call patients back who have had a fracture, but it was missed by the A&E doctor. Today that task was delegated to me.

The first report I got was from a lady of 65. She had fallen 10 days before, and had had an X-ray that showed a subtle but significant fracture. The junior doctor had missed it and told her that all was well. It was only today that the radiologist had reported it. I phoned her up and explained our mistake and got her to come back and get it plastered.

Far from being angry, she was apologetic about the trouble *she* had caused. Some people are just too nice for their own good. She explained that she had not come back as she didn't want to bother anyone. So she sat there, in obvious pain for 10 days, until she got my call.

Luckily, she didn't put a complaint in. If she had, I think the fault would not have been with the junior doctor but the system for taking so long for a radiologist to report an X-ray. We are soon having X-rays put on computers – why can't there be a radiologist on to do 'hot reporting' on the X-rays as soon as the X-ray is done? They wouldn't even need to leave their office to do this. At night, couldn't we have one radiologist up for a whole area hot reporting all the X-rays and CT scans done? (Or even sending the scan off to the other side of the world, where the time difference means it can be reported on immediately without having to wake up the radiologist?) This seems to me to be an efficient way of reporting urgent scans: it is safer for the patient and it is good education for all doctors.

Let's bring in reforms to the NHS; but sensible ones, ones that will help and make a difference. I think that this one might be a good idea.

Things have improved… but they need to be better still

For all the moans I have about A&E, some things have got better. Last night I was working and a patient came in with a dislocated shoulder. My junior colleague had never dealt with one before and had only seen them put back twice. I asked them to see the patient with me supervising the procedure. I asked my colleague how much sedation he wanted to give. The answer given was about three times as much as the patient should have received. If she had received that dose of analgesia, she could have had a respiratory complication (i.e. stopped breathing).

The answer given, though, was the dose I gave for a very similar patient about four years ago. Then I had little night supervision and the junior doctors just got on with it. We would be the ones seeing the sickest patients. There was a 'see one, do one, teach one' attitude. There was no senior A&E doctor on the 'shop floor' supervising me when I was doing nights. I don't know if any patients came to harm, but without senior supervision they could have.

Thankfully, because of the extra resources, there is more and more supervision of very junior doctors by middle-grade doctors like me. (We still could do with a bit more supervision from our bosses though.) However, some of my colleagues work in hospitals where it is not the case that there is always a middle-grade A&E doctor present on the shop floor. I think that this just isn't safe – if you are acutely unwell an experienced doctor, or a supervised junior one, not someone who is new to the job, should see you immediately. It is barmy that in this country that the sickest patients are frequently seen first by the most junior doctors, especially out of working hours.

If the resources were put into employing more senior doctors on the shop floor 24 hours a day, then patients would receive better care. The NHS would also save money in the long run as there would be fewer unnecessary admissions and good initial treatment is cheaper than expensive long-term care and lawsuits. The argument that there are not enough senior A&E doctors to provide 24-hour care is folly. If the specialty was made more attractive, and training jobs increased, then there would be enough to go round.

Harming yourself

I asked a psychiatrist to come down and see a patient who had taken 10 paracetamol and told me that if they were discharged from hospital they were going to kill themselves. This was her 15th attempted suicide in the last six months. She didn't seem too distressed by what she was saying, but I had to refer her.

The psychiatrist came down to see her. Luckily he knew her very well. Despite what she was saying he discharged her and said to me, 'She has got a personality disorder. By referring her to me you are encouraging her behaviour.' He then muttered quietly, 'Between you and me, she needs more friends and not more prescribed drugs – but I can't prescribe friends. But, hey, that's my job. I just hope I am right and she doesn't kill herself.' I chuckled as he went about writing his notes. It also made me think...

A great deal of the A&E workload is now seeing patients with suicide attempts. It is one of the most common reasons for youngsters (and the not so young) to be admitted to hospital. I don't know what it is – the increased stress of modern living? more and more stresses at school? or the prevalence of drugs? – but the numbers of attempted suicides seem to be rising.

Seeing a genuinely depressed patient is upsetting. They deserve your full attention and care as they are just as ill as anyone with a heart attack or broken bone but, as described above, a section of patients do take minor overdoses as a way of getting attention. Instead of being recognised as such they are now labelled as having a personality disorder. It can be very hard to make the distinction between people genuinely in need of help and those with a personality disorder (who also need help – but not by being referred as an emergency since that just gives positive feedback to their behaviour). I am just glad that I have got access to psychiatrists who can make that assessment for me.

There is also a large cohort of patients that comes in repeatedly after having self-harmed by cutting. It is hard to not be infuriated with them, especially when it is very busy, knowing that they caused their own problem. It is also hard to understand how someone could inflict so much pain and damage on themselves. However, they too need our attention and to dismiss them as time wasters is unfair. My eyes were opened to the problem last week, when a frequent cutter came back. As we were very quiet, I had time to chat with her, while suturing her wounds. She told me that she cut as a way of giving herself the control over her life that she had never had and that she had become addicted to it. She had been abused when younger and this was her way of coping. Again, A&E can only solve the acute problem. People like her need more help from other services.

ℒ Factitious behaviour

Some people come to A&E for bizarre reasons. I have seen two recently who have made up symptoms to get morphine or sympathy. The first I saw was a fantastic actress. She said that she had fallen off her bike. She was carrying her arm and wouldn't let me go near it, saying that she gets recurrent dislocations. She just kept on asking me for painkillers.

Dislocated shoulders can be agony, so I gave her some morphine and sent her for an X-ray. I asked her to wait while I arranged for someone to escort her to X-ray; however, as soon as my back was turned she got up and walked out of the hospital, ready for a night high on the morphine. Clever girl! She fooled me and made me feel like a right prat.

The next case was of a woman who pretended that she had HIV (human immunodeficiency virus) and had stopped taking her anti-retrovirals because of the side-effects. At the time I didn't realise she was lying because her story was so convincing. She claimed she was very short of breath and so I referred her to the medical team for treatment of an AIDS (acquired immunodeficiency syndrome)-related pneumonia. They were fooled as well. She was kept in and given expensive drugs for three days, by which time no-one could trace any old notes and her HIV test was negative. It's a weird world working in A&E.

ℒ People who work in the A&E department

There are lots of people who work in A&E – not just doctors and nurses. Here is a quick review of the people I spend my days with.

Emergency nurse practitioners (ENPs) – specially trained nurses who can treat minor injuries independently. They have taken a lot of the pressure off A&E doctors and done more for reducing waits in A&E than any other development. They write a lot of notes for each patient and can see fractures on X-rays (which I need a magnifying glass for) from 10 metres.

Pharmacists – go round improving doctors' spelling with green pens. Often save the arses of junior (and senior) doctors.

Receptionists – run the whole show. Know how to do everything. Massive amounts of common sense. I often think that if we sacked all the doctors and gave the receptionists a stethoscope, the NHS would be a better place. They keep the waiting masses in order with flair and frequently an iron rod.

Consultants – the senior doctors. Have years of experience and when they are on the shop floor, they make the place so much more efficient and patients get excellent treatment. Unfortunately, they are often in their offices answering complaints, or at meetings explaining why patients have 'breached' their 4-hour

126

rule (probably because the consultants were in a meeting explaining why other patients 'breached' as opposed to seeing patients)

Registrars/staff grade doctors/SpR doctors – below the consultants, more experienced than the SHOs. We are the ones who, when asked a question, will take off our glasses and put them in our mouths to look as if we have some intelligence and knowledge when really we are just playing for time.

SHOs/F2 – the junior rank of doctors working in A&E. Some are excellent. All are hard working – or forced to work hard by their appalling rotas which often mean that they work mostly unsocial shifts so that the more senior doctors can have a life. However, they only work for 4–6 months in the A&E department, so medical staffing planners can get away with it without too many complaints.

A&E secretary – she knows everything and everybody, does everything, finds everything and without her the place would fall apart. The most amazing organisational skills I have seen. This is not being sexist, but I don't think a man could ever replace our secretary – we can't multitask and she can.

Sisters – the lynchpins of A&E. They make sure that a 'shift' is run properly, coordinate the department along with the senior doctors, run the show, get paid bugger all and if they want promotion get pushed into management.

Charge nurses – male sisters. I call them brothers. They don't find it amusing except the vegetarian communist one, who keeps on trying to get me to join his commune.

Staff nurses – the work horses of the A&E. Usually excellent, but there are a few disgruntled and eccentric ones, especially the breed known as 'agency staff nurses'.

Health-care assistants – do the jobs nurses used to do, except give out drugs. Get paid a criminally small amount for such a vital job. It's a disgrace.

Physiotherapists – specialists in musculoskeletal problems. Female ones are usually very fit and male ones good at sport.

Occupational therapists – a cross between a social worker and a physiotherapist. Vital in helping elderly patients get out of A&E.

Radiographer – the person who does your X-rays. Not a doctor, but highly skilled and valuable members of the A&E team. Spend 3–4 years at university learning about human anatomy, physics and how to read doctors' writing.

Too posh to wash?

I was struggling at work today. The nurses on the 'shop floor' were flat out. I needed observations doing and drugs given, and neither was happening quickly. A patient had been calling out for 15 minutes for a commode before they got one. A patient needed changing from their wet incontinence pad, but it was left on for long enough to make the patient cry. Admittedly, we were busy, but the nursing care the patients were getting was not adequate, although there were nurses around. There were two ENPs, who now treat minor injuries. There was a specialist DVT (deep vein thrombosis) nurse seeing a patient as well. The urology nurse specialist had been asked to chat to a patient about their catheter and the cardiac specialist nurse was looking at an ECG and deciding if a patient needed to go to the coronary care unit.

I think all these jobs are valuable, and A&E would be lost without the input of specialist nurses, especially in the days of reduced doctor's hours. But is it right that we have so many nurse specialists when simple nursing procedures such as washing, doing observations, etc., are being left to a handful of overworked and underpaid junior nurses and nursing auxiliaries who have not got the time to do it properly.

You may think that it is the job of the senior sisters to organise the caring of the patients better. However, so much of their time is spent on managerial matters, planning meetings and worrying about targets, etc., that they have less and less clinical time to spend looking after patients and mentoring the junior nurses.

Often, the basic nursing tasks are performed by the nursing auxiliaries (health-care assistants). They, I believe, are the least appreciated and most valuable members of the A&E team. They do all the basic nursing tasks except give drugs. They take bloods, insert cannulas, do ECGs and, when time allows, they care for the patients. Last week I went to the leaving do of a health-care assistant of 10 years' experience. She had got a job at Tesco on the tills – earning more than her present job. But it wasn't just her leaving do: it was a joint one with an excellent senior A&E nurse who, because she wanted promotion and a pay rise, was pushed into a managerial role as a 'patient pathway coordinator' as opposed to nursing.

We need more nurses in nursing care. I am not saying we should cut the specialist nurses. I am just saying that we need more nurses employed to nurse… and they need better pay, both junior and senior, otherwise they will continue to leave the NHS or move into management and we need their skills where it really matters – on the shop floor.

How to lose a friend

I am good friends with some of the nurses at work, but I think that I have lost a friend today. She was chaperoning me doing a rectal examination. The patient had diarrhoea – I was checking that she (the patient not the nurse) didn't have something called overflow diarrhoea, where severe constipation only lets liquid faeces pass the blockage. I examined her and my suspicions were confirmed. As I withdrew my gloved finger, I examined it and saw lots of diarrhoea. As I took the gloves off, the elastic of the gloves acquired a life of their own. It then all happened in slow motion. I saw particles of faeces fly off my glove straight onto my colleague's uniform, leaving a brown splatter pattern right over her left breast. 'Ooops! I am sorry' didn't appear to be sufficient and I found myself cleaning a lot of commodes that night.

Hero to heroin

The ambulance call came through; '21-year-old male. Unconscious, respiration rate 5. Having to be bagged (artificially ventilated) by the paramedics. IVDU – intravenous drug user'.

It was the third similar patient this week. I met the ambulance as it arrived and we wheeled him into Resus. Behind came a distraught mother and father. We went through the basic treatment of the unconscious patient. The ambulance man continued to keep him alive by giving him oxygen. I examined him and tried to get a cannula in. It was virtually impossible: all his veins had scarred up from excessive use in injecting drugs. I eventually managed to find one in his neck.

I could now give him the reversal for heroin – naloxone. I was only a relatively naive junior doctor at this stage, with a limited experience of heroin overdoses. I gave him the full dose of reversal medication. It blocks the morphine receptors, and means that the patient quickly wakes up, starts to breathe for himself and comes down off his high. ...And he did. In about 3 minutes he had woken up, pulled his Guedel airway (piece of equipment used to keep the airway open in an unconscious patient and let them breathe) out of his mouth and started to shout and curse.

'What the f**k did you do that for, you bastard?'

I tried to explain that his mum had called an ambulance and he had needed the paramedics to keep him alive. I expected him to be grateful. As I said, I was naive to the gratitude of some patients.

'You can f**k off. I am out of here.' He pulled off his ECG monitor and cannula and stormed out, looking for another fix.

Heroin has powerful qualities. It makes the user fixate only on the drug and nothing else matters. They ignore all else in the search for the ultimate 'nirvana' high. No need, therefore, for the social niceties of being pleasant to hospital staff and the paramedics who saved his life. No need to show love to his parents. No need to conform to accepted social standards and so it is no wonder many steal from grannies or take excessive risks as prostitutes to pay for the drug. There is just the need to get that high and so he left looking for a hit again.

The danger of what I did was that the reversal wears off quicker than the heroin, so he may have gone back to his unconscious state. Also, with him in the plucking/cold turkey state he could be a danger to himself and staff. I learned my lesson: give very small doses of the reversal slowly over time, so they are too drowsy to up and leave.

As he left I had a word with his distraught parents. They had been loving parents but he had got in with the wrong crowd. He used to be a footballer – apparently quite promising. He was a hero for his school's team, being top scorer for three years, but then the wrong crowd came along. He had started with cannabis and then moved onto ecstasy, cocaine and then heroin. He was in and out of prison and then either on the streets or kipping at various friends' houses. He paid for his fixes with petty crime. He had been on a methadone treatment programme (methadone is a heroin substitute, but does not give the same high) but it hadn't worked. He had been loving as a child and now they described him as a monster that they didn't recognise. They loved him, but hated who he had become.

At this point in my career, I was new to drug abusers and the thing that I found most strange (which shows that I obviously have deep middle-class misconceptions and prejudices) was that they seemed a normal loving middle-class parents. His mother was a nursery nurse and his father was a taxi driver. They were not alcoholics and they had not abused him or neglected him. It just shows that drugs can affect anyone, no matter what their upbringing.

They asked what they could do. I didn't have the answer. The police were failing him. The social services were failing and so were the methadone programmes – he still went out and took heroin. He might die soon after another overdose, and they and I felt helpless. That week, three similar patients had come in. The police also said that another had died before an ambulance had been called. Apparently, a new drug dealer was on the street and was selling a stronger version of heroin. It was getting people more and more addicted and killing some of them because of overdoses as a result of its strength. The policeman told me that they needed to catch this dealer quickly or there would be more deaths. His colleague joked that at least the crime rate would go down if he wasn't caught... but it wasn't funny. These addicts are people's sons, daughters, fathers and mothers. They also have potential to be reintegrated into society and to become assets to the country. We are failing them as much as they are failing themselves and their families.

So could anything be done? Well, possibly. A couple of years after I saw this patient, the government brought in some pilot schemes, some of which are using the experience of the Swiss authorities, who have made heroin free and available to use on prescription in special clinics run by specialists. The patients can go twice a day and get their normal fix, but with a standardised drug so that they don't overdose. It is a clean and safe environment. The users no longer go to the dealers as free heroin is available from the clinics. Crime is down, as they no longer need to mug grannies to pay for their fixes. Dealers have left because of market forces and so fewer kids are starting heroin. The users are medicalised, the glamour of drug-taking is reduced and their lives have been stabilised. They can start to get jobs and when they are ready they can be transferred to methadone and slowly weaned off the drug.

It is a possible solution. But it is controversial because the government is, in effect, saying to people that taking heroin is no longer a crime – come round and have some of our free stuff. However, initial results show that this approach works. I think it is controversial not to consider this scheme. It is just a shame for the user I saw and his family that he does not live in one of the trial areas.

Taking the piss

Life can be a bit unfair for patients. If you sit quietly, then you usually don't get pushed to the front of the queue, but if you make a fuss sometimes your care is speeded up. Today I learned that if you piss on the floor you'll get seen straight away.

The 'minors' nurse asked if I could see a patient because he wanted him out of the department ASAP. He explained:

'You'll know him. He is a regular. He's completely well and a bit of a pain in the rear (he may have been slightly more fruity in his description). Get rid of him… Oh, and he has just pissed all over the floor and is swearing at us.'

The nurse was right. I knew him very well. He was an alcoholic (not a particularly pleasant alcoholic either) who had turned down help dozens of times. He usually came in when a member of the public saw him comatose and called an ambulance.

'Hello sir. You seemed to have urinated all over the floor. Is everything OK?' I enquired.

'I couldn't be bothered to walk to the toilet,' he slurred.

'A pleasure to see you, sir. Always a pleasure. Do you want to sit in the chair?' I asked (he was standing and looking a little threatening).

The nurse interjected: 'He has pissed on that as well.'

'Well, sir, I suggest we do this consultation somewhere else… why don't you move away from the pool of urine beneath your legs and come with me to the next cubicle? Why are you here?'

'Don't know. I was having a kip and them bastards in green brought me in.'

'They are ambulance men, sir. Not in any way do you know their parentage. And please don't swear.' I was losing my patience but also quite enjoying the amusement this patient was giving me. I added, 'Are you unwell? Have you banged your head?'

He showed me his arm. He needed to be here because he had a laceration that needed suturing. I explained that to him, went into the theatre to open up all the expensive suturing packs and called for him. But he had left – probably back to the pub or the nearest park bench to finish the kip that had been so rudely interrupted. Oh well… on to the next patient. I'm sure he'll be back.

Off on holiday

Yipeee… I am off on holiday! No work for two weeks. I can leave it all behind and not have to think about anything but sun, sea, sand and trying to persuade my wife to have sex.

We were flying in economy class to Dubai – to sample everyone's favourite new tourist destination. In an attempt to impress my wife, I hadn't bought a paper and had planned to try and charm her en route and therefore guarantee the fourth 's'.

'Stop boring me. I am trying to sleep,' she responded, with no flick of the hair or any sign that I was guaranteed a holiday shag on arrival. She fell asleep and I had no paper to read on the journey. I was shit bored.

An hour later she was still asleep and I was still bored.

Two hours later she was still asleep and I was trying to play noughts and crosses with myself.

Then relief! The scariest thing you can hear if you are a doctor on a plane (except perhaps 'We have hijacked your plane, etc.' – that is probably scarier): 'Is there a doctor on board?' I was so bored that I jumped up and went running. I wasn't thinking what could be wrong, I was thinking, 'Will I get an upgrade with some better films to watch?'

I got there and saw a woman in her 50s totally unconscious. Oh shit! I couldn't wake her. I was no longer concerned about the upgrade – as long as they could give me change of pants at the end of this I would be OK. I went through basic first aid – ABC. A for airway – that was OK. She was still breathing and she still had a pulse. OK, she is safe for a minute – but what do I do now? I asked questions, getting more frantic.

'Does anyone know her? Who is with her? Did she fit?' No one knew her. Shit! It is easy in a resuscitation department, but at 12 000 feet a little less so.

Think, Edwards, think. The algorithm that all emergency doctors remember is ABCDEFG and the DEFG, stands for don't ever forget glucose. I turned round and said, 'Can anyone do a BM?' (sugar level test).

What the hell was I saying – we were in aeroplane aisle and not an A&E. Why didn't I ask for a CT scan, a 'chem. 20' or an ECG? I obviously got blank looks from the passengers around me that I had hoped had mysteriously turned into nurses.

I asked to see what was in their emergency bag. At the same time, the pilot asked if he should divert. I had one lady's well-being in my hands and 300 people's holiday at stake, including my own. This was not part of the relaxing holiday plan.

Bingo! In the emergency drug box, I saw they had glucagon. It reverses the effects of insulin and can increase your sugar level. I might as well give it a go, I thought. I opened the pack and then realised that in the last five years of medicine I hadn't given an injection. I was on my own and so gave it a go.

A minute or two later, she started to wake up. Yes, it was working. 'Get her some sugar,' I called out. About five stewardesses came running forward (which was a beautiful, wonderful vision). I got more sugar than you could wish for. I gave it to her and she became coherent. It turned out she was a diabetic, had taken her insulin and then got drunk as she was scared of flying. She then felt sick and so didn't eat any dinner. Her glucose level had dropped dangerously low and she had therefore become unconscious. The treatment had taken about 30 minutes of my time, broken up the journey, stopped her getting sick and prevented my holiday plane being diverted.

The senior steward approached me. 'Thank you so much – please let me upgrade you for the rest of the journey' Lovely jubbly – I thought. I'll be mixing with millionaires. I went and got my wife, who was a little embarrassed at the fuss.

With free drinks flowing, I got horny and she got… tired and fell back to sleep. At least I now had a free paper to read while she was asleep. Being the aeroplane saviour also got me appreciated by her when we finally arrived in a hotel.

You can't escape from the job of being a doctor, but it does have its advantages…

Hospital inefficiencies

It was 1 a.m. and I was knackered. It was ridiculously busy. It had been non-stop for the last 5 hours. I was examining a little old lady who had fallen and broken her wrist and it needed manipulation (pulling back into a better position). This is a very common A&E procedure and I was getting ready to manipulate this woman's arm when the 'red phone' went off. A heart attack was coming in, in 3 minutes' time.

I had no option but to postpone the woman's manipulation and make her wait at least another hour. I apologised that there were only two doctors for the whole of A&E and that she would have to wait. I also explained to the other people waiting how busy we were. There were a few moans and groans, a couple of patients self-discharged but no-one seemed that annoyed and most seemed to understand.

However, it didn't need to be that way. There were only two A&E doctors working, but there were lots of other doctors in the hospital who could have come and helped. However, there isn't always the cooperation between A&E and the specialist doctors based in the rest of the hospital. If A&E is busy, then there is no arrangement for them to come down just when we need an extra pair of hands (as opposed to see an admission or give specialist advice).

So there I am, slogging my guts out, while others are sitting in the doctors' mess less than 200 metres away. It doesn't often happen that we are the only doctors working (in addition to the medical doctors – they are always as busy as us), but it does happen frequently enough to warrant making plans on how to utilise all the doctors at night. Being honest, the problem is that there are no expectations for the specialists to help out. When I was working as a specialist junior doctor, I would sit in the mess (even though I had A&E experience) while patients would wait to see an A&E doctor, because that is the way hospitals work.

It may seem a crazy reality, but it is how hospitals function at night. You wait 3 hours with a broken bone to see an A&E doctor, when there may have been an orthopaedic doctor sitting there doing nothing.

I think the reason that there is a tradition for specialist doctors to not come down and help 'just to lend a pair of hands' is because of the tradition of 24- to 48-hour shifts when these doctors needed to sleep. But this is no longer the case.

Nowadays, the vast majority of doctors only do 12-hour shifts and so can work through the whole of the shift.

There can also be a 'them and us' attitude between A&E and specialist doctors. Just because we are the ones who provide the rest of the hospital with a lot of their workload, this shouldn't make us the enemy. The other reason for this lack of collaboration is that some A&E doctors don't want other specialist doctors 'stepping on our toes' and coming in and managing the cases that we can deal with. Surely, what is important is not which part of the hospital micromanagement the doctor works for, but what their skills are and whether they are appropriately trained to see the patient.

Reforms are a necessity for the NHS. Hospitals are starting to introduce a hospital-at-night scheme, where doctors cooperate more, but it doesn't usually involve the A&E doctors – what madness. We need better reforms which break the inertia of senior management and improve the cooperation between A&E doctors and specialists. This is one example where I think real change to practice would make a massive difference. (And it did.)

One month later, I was doing another set of nights when a friend of mine was the orthopaedic doctor on for the hospital for a week of nights. She realised how busy we were and spent the whole night (when she could have been asleep) helping out by seeing patients who obviously had an orthopaedic problem directly – as opposed to them seeing an A&E doctor first. It made a massive difference, but led to complaints from her colleagues that it set a 'precedent'. How sad that working together can be frowned upon by some of our colleagues.

Crying wolf

All A&Es get their 'regulars'. Often they are homeless people, or drunks or drug addicts. They attend frequently, as their life styles mean that they are prone to getting ill. Also, they don't know how to access primary care resources, or perhaps choose not to. Some staff can get quite close to these patients. It leads to a dangerous relationship, whereby whenever they want shelter or food they attend A&E, as opposed to going through other more appropriate channels.

My colleague saw one of our regulars yesterday. It was his 145th attendance in three years. He comes when he needs a wash or food and shelter. He always puts on a fake abdominal pain and trades getting his needs catered for in return for not making a fuss and leaving soon after dinner. He came in again with abdominal pain, this time after a supposed fight. A brief examination resulted in the usual general tenderness in the stomach. My colleague told him that A&E was not the right place for him to go to when he wanted food and he was discharged without being given dinner. He protested but everyone assumed it was because of the lack of food.

The next day he came back with a ruptured spleen from the fight. He was rushed to theatre and, thankfully, is making a good recovery after two days in the high-dependency ward. My colleague feels awful. But I think some of the blame lies with the patient for crying wolf and with all of the A&E staff for in the past positively reinforcing his wolf-crying behaviour.

P.S. Three weeks after he was discharged he was back in A&E

with abdominal pain. He was given food and left. However, for the last few months he has not been to A&E. Apparently he is currently in jail. As soon as he is out, he will be back. He needs social services, police and A&E to come up with a joined-up plan for him. He also needs to stop crying wolf.

Blind to the problems

It was 4 p.m. and a panicked 29-year-old builder walked in. He had had a sudden clouding of vision over his left eye. The other thing I also noticed was that he was overweight... very overweight. He made John Prescott seem svelte. I examined him and took a history from him. He was reasonably well, but admitted to a poor diet and little exercise. I looked in his eye and there was evidence of damage done to the back of the eye by diabetes. I then did a sugar test – 18 – very high, virtually confirming a diagnosis of diabetes. I explained what I thought was going on, and referred him urgently to the eye clinic and then via his GP to the diabetologists. For me, it was a simple case. But for him, it is the start of a life with the miserable potential complications of diabetes: eye problems, heart disease, nerve damage and kidney disease. What was interesting in this case was his age.

There are two types of diabetes mellitus. Type 1 is the type children get when (possibly) an autoimmune disease damages the pancreas, which then stops the production of insulin. Insulin is a hormone that is produced after eating to lower the blood sugar level and store this ingested energy. Too high a level of sugar in the bloodstream damages fragile tissues such as in

142

the back of the eyes, the kidneys and the body's blood vessels. Type 2 diabetes is a problem with the body's metabolism and sensitivity to insulin and usually occurs in the later part of life (if you have a genetic predisposition for it). However, if by overeating you have already had a lifetime's metabolism when you are young, then you can actually get it at a young age.

This is what had happened to this patient of mine. Overeating and under-exercising had caused him to have a much older person's illness. Unless he massively changes his lifestyle, he will get all the consequences described above, retire early and get his money's worth (and yours) from the NHS.

However, he isn't unique. The text books I first had when studying said you couldn't make the diagnosis below the age of 40, but I have seen him and three other people in their late 20s/early 30s with type 2 diabetes, and so have my colleagues. Amazingly, paediatric colleagues have seen this condition in teenagers. All of them have the disease at so young an age as a result of obesity.

Obesity not only contributes to the diabetic epidemic, being overweight makes one more likely to get cancer, heart disease, stroke, breathing difficulties and osteoarthritis. It is a ticking time bomb for health. The fact that one in three youngsters are overweight makes it an epidemic waiting to happen – an epidemic that I believe could be a real threat to the viability of the NHS.

When I was at school, nobody seemed to care. Maggie Thatcher sold off my school's playing field and privatised the school canteen and then they sold shit food for a profit. Also, I wasn't taught cooking, and if it wasn't for my wife (a wonderful cook), then the local curry house owner (also a wonderful cook) and 'pizza a go-go' would have much larger profits. Up until Jamie Oliver kicked up a fuss, Blair didn't seem that bothered. However, things are changing, but not really quickly enough.

Why not slap on a 20 per cent shit food tax (with qualified nutritionists deciding what is unhealthy) and use the money to give out healthy food vouchers with child support benefit? Why not ban junk food advertising before the 9 p.m. watershed and not just around kids' TV programmes? Why not stop kids leaving schools at lunchtime so they can't eat crap from the local newsagent? Why not put proper amounts of money into a cycling network as opposed to painting a bit of pavement and then producing leaflets saying how much you have done? Whatever the arguments are against these proposals, then surely the fact that if we don't do something our nation's health will be buggered in the future is a decent enough counter argument.

It needs a change of mind-set from the government, not just tweaking around the edges. Prevention is much better than cure and in the long run cheaper, but until they do something then we are faced with the problem. Individually, people must make an effort and medical staff must encourage them to make an effort.

Finally, if we did as a nation lose weight, then it would not be so embarrassing when I go abroad and see a group of men sunbathing on the beach, where the Spanish life guards and World Wildlife Federation volunteers try to roll them back into the sea…

It is also a sobering thought, that however many years I work in A&E, I will never make as much impact on people's health as Jamie Oliver will... and I don't even cook as well as him... or earn as much... or sell as many books... or say 'pukka' as authentically.

When patients make jokes

The last few days at work, I have noticed an increasing number of very poor jokes coming from patients. It is getting to epidemic proportions. Please stop. I have heard them all before. I like new jokes, so learn some before coming to A&E but please don't use any of the ones below that I have heard in the last two days.

Dr: 'What brought you in?'.
Patient: 'An ambulance'.

Dr: 'How do you feel?'.
Patient: 'With my hands. How do you feel?'

When taking blood. Patient: 'Ho-ho-ho it's the vampires.'

Yesterday, a woman who works in Asda came in with the worst possible dress sense and one of the worst jokes:

'Any allergies?'
'Only hospitals... ha ha ha'.

'So', I thought, 'I have heard that joke a thousand times. Let me laugh, if I find it funny, but please don't laugh on my behalf.'

However, I got her back. I went shopping to Asda that evening. I paid with a large note, put the change in my back pocket and tapped my back pocket twice. How I laughed. She thought: 'I have heard that joke a thousand times. Let me laugh, if I find it funny, but please don't laugh on my behalf'.

Seriously though, there is nothing better than having a bit of banter with your patients at work. It makes my day so much more enjoyable. So although I have heard those jokes before, on second thoughts keep them coming.

Ooops again

Blaming tiredness was no excuse. Blaming lack of experience was also not an excuse. I genuinely mucked up but luckily the patient didn't complain. He was a 90-year-old war hero – he had won a VC in WW2. He had tripped and got a cut to his forearm which needed stitching.

It was at the beginning of my working life and I was still keen to suture. Now I find it very time-consuming and usually delegate it to the nurses, but at that point in my training I found it really satisfying. I cleaned the area thoroughly. I then sterilised the wound with some Betadine (antiseptic wash) then opened my sutures and slowly and methodically put in 10 stitches. The wound closed easily and I was proud of the cosmetic appearance.

'There we go, sir,' I said. 'Not a bad job if I may say so myself.'

He looked at it in a satisfied way. 'Should I go to my practice nurse to get the stitches removed?' he asked.

'Yes, in seven days. Take care now… '

He picked up his stuff and then took five steps away and came back to me. 'Is it normal to not use local anaesthetic nowadays?' he asked.

I thought he was joking and then I realised that I had completely forgot to use it. WHAT THE HELL! I had forgotten to put in local anaesthetic, and he had been too polite to tell me. Oh my God! I'll get the sack. The pain he must have felt! I went white and then nearly cried.

'I am so, so sorry…' I started to confide in him. 'I have been so stressed recently. It's my first A&E job and I just seem to find it all so stressful. I don't know what I was thinking. I am so sorry.'

My eyes started to well up and my bottom lip quivered.

'Don't worry. It didn't hurt that much. It was nothing when you have been fired at on the Normandy beaches. You're a good doctor – don't get stressed by one mistake.'

He was so nice.

'I only asked because I wanted to know if it had become normal practice.'

He left and I went to cry for a minute or two. I don't know why this encounter had made me cry – perhaps it was just the stress of the last four months coming out.

Two weeks letter he sent a letter to the hospital. He thanked me personally for a 'pleasant and pain-free visit to the A&E department'. Thank God for patients like him.

More inefficiencies of hospital care

Despite what you see on TV, most cases coming to A&E are what are termed 'medical' cases, such as chest infections, chest pain and little old ladies with a 'collapse – ?cause'.

Last night I had a large number of medical cases come to A&E. Some I sent home, but quite a few needed admission into hospital for in-patient care. These patients are called 'medical referrals'. Although they are seen and stabilised by the A&E doctors, they need to be referred to the medical doctors for admission and continuing care. The medical team of doctors is generally the busiest specialty in the hospital and in a medium-sized hospital will often admit over 30 patients in a 24-hour period.

As it routinely takes over an hour to properly sort out a new sick patient and write up their notes, not to mention catch up on the routine day-to-day jobs, you can see why they are so busy. Once I have referred a patient to them, it can often take several hours before the patient is reviewed by a member of the medical team and a final plan of action made. This means that the more I can do in A&E to diagnose, treat and manage the patient, the better and faster it is for everyone concerned. However with the 4-hour target and the lack of staff compared with patients, this is often very difficult to do.

Last night the A&E SHO and I were working flat out all night. So were the medical team of doctors. Because we were so busy, sick patients were waiting about 2 hours to see us (the A&E team) and then about another 3 hours to see the medical team (if they needed to). Despite everyone's best efforts, I don't think that as a hospital we provided that good a service that night.

Many of the patients I saw had quite simple problems that, although needing admission, were very easy to treat and construct a management plan for. However, once they had seen me and been referred to the medical team, the hospital policy is that they are then 'reclerked' by the medical team. Re-clerking means that all the same questions that I had already asked are repeated and a full examination is performed again. The results of this re-clerking are then written down on hospital paper as opposed to the separate A&E notes where I had written the exact same things several hours earlier. For the busy medics, this is a complete waste of time. Especially so, as one of the medical doctors reviewing the patients that I had referred used to work with me as one of my juniors and has a lot less medical experience than I do.

Now, I do agree that it is good for patients to be reviewed by the team they are coming in under, and it is vital that important questions are clarified and important parts of the examination rechecked. But why do they need to do a time-consuming rewriting of their notes? Sometimes it is necessary if the A&E team have been so busy that the patient might not have been properly sorted out before referral, but often this is not the case. Because of pointless hospital rules, the notes are simply copied out by the medical specialists from the A&E doctors' notes. Haven't we heard of a photocopier and then writing: 'In addition:...? '

As well as being inefficient, the system is demoralising. The medical doctors have not trained as doctors simply to repeat someone else's work and the A&E doctors get annoyed as they think, 'What is the point of me writing all those notes if they are just going to get re-written?'. What is needed is a single 'tier' of care. Who that initial doctor is, is not that important. The only thing that is important is that the doctor treating the patient has had sufficient skills and supervision. The skills to treat 'medically' ill patients are something both A&E and medical doctors should have. There should then be a system in place for handing over the care of the patient to the inpatient team, who then appropriately review them closely.

There are two ways of bringing about changes that I believe are needed to improve care and improve efficiency. The first route is what some smaller hospitals are starting to do when they are 'down grading' their A&E department. Instead of having A&E doctors see patients, a triage nurse sees them and then asks the appropriate specialist doctor to see them straight off. In principle, this is fine. It gets rid of the inefficiencies of 'double clerking'. It is also a model that can be used in areas of the country where there is not a large cohort of experience emergency doctors. However, I think that this is a poor solution. The A&E doctors have a specific interest, training and skills in emergency medicine. If you come in with an acute problem then we are the right people to see you initially and give you immediate care – especially if the cause of why you are unwell is not easily identifiable by the triage nurse (e.g. being unconscious could have a surgical cause, medical cause or be the result of trauma). Also, properly trained A&E doctors are particularly good at preventing patients who do not need admission from being admitted unnecessarily. They are also very good at treating the sickest of patients who do need admission.

For all those reasons, I think that A&E doctors are the ones who should see the patients initially. But we need sufficient resources so that we can spend time with our sick patients and we need to not be constrained by targets of getting them out of A&E ASAP. Once referred to the medical team they should be reviewed by medical doctors with a specific interest in acute problems – called acute physicians. In the UK we have started to increase the number of acute physicians, which is fantastic for patient care as they have the specialist skills in caring for very sick patients in the first 48 hours of their admission and, if appropriate, organizing speedy discharge.

There is a system in Australia where patients stay under the A&E team for a lot longer and it works very well. However, they have a greater number of A&E doctors than we do in the UK and so have the manpower to properly sort out their patients before passing them on to the specialist doctors. We are not going to suddenly triple the number of A&E doctors overnight so we need to think about how things can be improved currently.

What we need to do is improve the integration of the A&E teams and medical teams. For example, an A&E doctor could assess the patient and, if necessary, admit them to the acute ward with a management plan and drug chart written up. This would happen without the need for a medical doctor to repeat the whole process. They would then be handed over to the medical team on call who could review the patient without repeating all the notes. The medics would therefore have a lot more time available and could come down to A&E and see patients directly (i.e. instead of their being seen by A&E doctors first) as well as the other admissions such as those that are referred directly from GPs. This would also mean that A&E doctors would have more time to sort out their patients properly and do a 'good clerking' which doesn't need redoing by the medical doctors.

To bring in this mind-set of changes of managing acute medical patients would require doctors of different specialties (A&E, Acute Medics and 'General Medics') to work together and trust each other. People then need to realise that what is important is how well the patient is being treated and not which particular specialty the doctor seeing them works for.

I hope that these changes get brought in and that I can just get on with my job – looking after sick patients who have not had to endure long waits to see me. I don't want to have to move to Australia to get job satisfaction. I want things to change over here.

P.S. Mum, if you are reading this, don't worry, I wouldn't really move to Australia – I'll stay here and just rant after work instead.

Sad request for a MAP

The computer showed that the next patient was 'requesting MAP'. The medical student shadowing me believed me when I told him that as we were becoming a 'foundation hospital', one of our hospital's money-making mechanisms was giving out directions to lost people. I explained that we were in partnership with the AA and charged only £1.50 per direction. I was baffled when he muttered that he thought it was a good idea and could he come and watch how to give out appropriate advice. I shook my head, distressed that sarcasm had been taken off the medical school curriculum and replaced with bum licking. I went in the cubicle and started to ask the patient about her request for the morning-after pill – MAP.

She came with her husband and three-year-old child. She told me that the condom had split and therefore she needed the morning-after pill. They were holding hands and looked like a perfect couple. As I was going through how to take the pill, she burst into tears.

'But I want another baby. And I want to give my little one a brother or sister,' she said tearfully.

I asked why she had come for a morning-after pill then. I was being stupid and naive and she quite rightly told me so.

'It's all right for you. What with your good salary and three-bed semi. But we are struggling to pay the mortgage on our two-bedroom flat. My hubby is a Postie and we rely on my wage to pay the bills. I can't afford to go on maternity. We can't afford another baby. I want one, but can't have one. Give me the pill and don't ask questions please.'

I gave her the MAP and all the advice it entails. I couldn't really respond to her distress. I have the benefits of a good job and decent pay-packet (a terraced house though not semi-detached). For me, poverty and how people cope or don't with it, is something I see at work, but which doesn't ever enter my private life. I am so lucky and this encounter made me realise that.

P.S. I don't want this book to be burdened with patient advice, but please realise that the morning-after pill is a truly shit name. It is best used asap, but is still effective for up to three days. End of lecture.

Teaching

I love teaching medical students and medical students usually love coming to A&E as there is much to see and learn. But today I hated it. I had a third-year shadow me for a taster day in A&E. He was the most arrogant, pompous little shit I have ever met. He was rude to the patients and just tried to question my management in front of them. He had no ability to empathise with patients and viewed them solely as an illness entity and not a patient with an illness. I know he is only a third-year, but I would hate to be his patient if these personality traits are not knocked out of him.

I know when I first started medical school, not everyone was interviewed – some places were offered on the basis of exams alone. It is becoming academically harder and harder to get into medical school. However, you don't have to be a brain surgeon to be a doctor (you do have to be a doctor to be a brain surgeon though). What is needed is common sense and courtesy, not four As at A-level. I don't know what the interview process is like nowadays but I have some worries after trying to teach my student today.

Sorry, there was no real point to this story, I was just expressing my frustration.

ℒ₀ Even more hospital inefficiencies

We are massively in debt as a hospital and there are plans for a freeze on recruitment. It is not just redundancies in the NHS we have to worry about, but newly qualified nurses and physiotherapists, etc., not getting jobs. Apparently, this is because as a 'Trust' we are short of pennies.

I was feeling in a reflective mood, so on my break I went for a walk around the hospital. Through every corridor loads of the windows were open but below these windows were radiators pumping out hot air paid for by our taxes. I then went to see a friend on a ward. After meal time, plate upon plate of food was thrown away. Not necessarily because it was no good, but because there was no-one there feeding the patients; what a waste of money. I then wandered to the car park, and there were two parking attendants just sitting there, chatting, not really doing much – at our expense.

I walked past theatres and there were surgeons doing bugger all, because there were no beds for their patients to go to after surgery, and so their lists were cancelled. I walked back to the wards and saw that tests were being repeated because results had got lost through not being stored electronically.

I then saw patients being unnecessarily admitted to wards because of targets... and other patients who were sicker and costing the NHS more because they didn't get 'gold standard' treatment from the NHS earlier in their hospital stay. Then I went to A&E and saw doctors repeating each other's work.

I then carried on my wanderings. I accidentally went to the management suite. It was late in the evening and no-one was working there – but all the lights were on. Couldn't anyone turn them off? What are all these offices for? We need managers, but this many?

NHS money is being wasted left, right and centre. The NHS needs a bigger pot (especially emergency services), but the pot needs to be used a bit more sensibly. Quite rightly, the government wants to improve efficiency. It is just a shame they are doing it in such a bad way.

A weird rash

Last week I saw something I have never seen before. A child came in with a weird-looking rash that I didn't recognise. I asked my colleagues – they had no idea either. Then the paediatric doctor had a look, she was clueless. Finally, the senior consultant came to review.

'Do you read the newspapers?' he asked the mother.

'No. Why?' she responded, a bit perplexed.

'Your child has measles. You may have believed the stuff they said about MMR (measles, mumps and rubella). That's why I asked. Did he have the MMR?'

He hadn't. Mum had listened to some ridiculous stories perpetuated by the headline-seeking gutter press. As a result he hadn't been immunised. But he was lucky and OK to go home.

Today, I saw a much sadder case; a little girl who had also got measles. I recognised it now. But she was much sicker. She had to go to the paediatric intensive care ward. Her life was at risk as the virus had caused infection to the brain and she might suffer brain damage as a result. Her mum had also stopped her from having MMR, and was paying privately for single-injection immunisations, but her daughter hadn't had the measles one yet.

Measles is a serious killer (mumps and rubella aren't so good either). The MMR vaccination is not this evil autism-inducing injection that the media sometimes make us think. There is no evidence that it causes autism. However, there is evidence that if your child doesn't have the injection, they are at higher risk of getting these illnesses. Today I saw a child I shouldn't have. Have a proper think before you refuse your health visitor's advice.

Feeling guilty

Have you ever felt that you have contributed inadvertently to someone's demise? I have and I can't stop feeling guilty about it. It happened two days ago, and I have felt really shit since. He was a 45-year-old – a lovely bloke who came in reluctantly with his wife. Quite poignantly he explained that he didn't want to come in as 'you never get out of hospitals ok'.

He had had some chest discomfort after dinner. He thought it was indigestion. His wife wasn't so sure. She had seen posters advising you to call an ambulance if you had odd chest pains and this pain seemed to be getting worse. She (very sensibly) called 999. He was having a heart attack. The ambulance blue lighted him in, and I met him in the Resus department.

His ECG confirmed the diagnosis. The treatment for this (in our hospital, out of working hours) is a clot-busting drug. It is a very effective drug in these situations and opens up the artery that has become blocked. I have given it successfully many times in the past but there can be some rare but serious side-effects. One is bleeding in the brain. I took him and his wife through the risks and benefits in his case. I said it was low risk and that I had personally never had a problem.

We started the drug. Very quickly his speech became slurred. I stopped the drug straight away. Then he couldn't move the right side of his body and then he became unconscious. The drug had caused a bleed in his brain and he will suffer severe lifelong side-effects from the drug we injected. Although, medically, I did nothing wrong, and know that it was the right drug for his condition, I still feel guilty that I may have inadvertently contributed to his demise by giving him a drug that should have saved his life, not left him disabled for life. I find that hard to deal with.

Being called at home

I got a call from one of the nurses at home today. She sounded worried.

'I just thought I'd call you before one of the bosses. I think you need to know.' She sounded worried. 'Do you remember the old lady you treated yesterday? The lady with the very fast heart rate?'

I did. I was really pleased about how I had treated her. I had taken her and her son into the resuscitation bay and spent about 1 hour sorting her out properly. I had spent the whole time explaining to her and her son what we were doing and why. They commented on how nice we had been and how she was pleased that nowadays doctors aren't 'stuffy' and take the time to explain to them what we were doing. She also said how much more comfortable she felt that I had introduced myself as Nick as opposed to Dr Edwards.

'Yes I do. What's the matter?' I asked.

'Her son has sent a formal letter to the chief executive and as I was the nurse working with you I have been asked to comment.'

'What the hell. I thought... '

'The letter went on about your informal style and relaxed attitude. It talked about letting relatives into Resus and being present the whole time during a difficult and scary time.'

'But I thought they were happy with us,' I responded as I started to panic about such a formal complaint.

'I have got to go now. There is a long wait in minors. Bye. I'll phone back soon.'

She hung up before I could find out who I needed to speak to.

Oh my God! Why had they complained? What had I done? What was going to happen to me? I felt faint with anxiety. Very soon I was going to need A&E treatment for my own fast heart rate. Five minutes later she phoned back.

'As I was saying, the letter praised the entire department for being so wonderful and the family has given us a case of wine to say thank you! Well done.'

Getting thank you letters really does make work a pleasure. So does practical jokes and being wound up... but only after the event. If she is reading this, then I just want you to know that he who laughs last laughs loudest. Watch out...

Complaint letters

One of the most upsetting things for a doctor or a nurse is getting a complaint letter. We are human and sometimes we fall below the expected standard – then a complaint is justified. However, many complaints are preventable and caused by poor communication. The complaints which are upsetting are the unjustified ones and the ones sent out of a desire to seek compensation. The stresses of complaints are enormous. Your clinical skills are brought into question. Your name can appear in the local press, where everyone assumes you are guilty. Then there is the concern that it may affect your career as well as the personal feeling that you may have let people down.

Some legal complaints are utter bollocks, but often the hospital 'pays up' because the cost of the claim is cheaper than going to court against a 'no-win, no-fee' company.

What prompted me to write about complaints is one I received last week and I have been fuming about it ever since. I had seen a really sick and unwell asthmatic mother of three. She was 38. She had been into ICU twice in the past with breathing difficulties. She came in very unwell. I was really pleased with my very swift and good treatment. After the treatment in A&E, she was well enough to go to a normal ward as opposed to ICU. I really felt that we had saved her life.

When she was a bit better, I went and had a longer chat with her. She told me she that still smoked. I couldn't believe it. She had a life-threatening respiratory problem and still smoked. I told her, in no uncertain terms, that she was putting her children at risk of losing their mother. I told her it was

160

easier for her to give up smoking than for her partner to bring up their children alone. The whole time I was being polite and had her interests at heart. It would have been much easier to not give out advice.

I thought I had done the right thing. Apparently, I hadn't. She left hospital a week later and two months later she contacted the hospital. It wasn't to send us a thank you letter. She had called up the patient advocacy team. They had written a complaint on her behalf. I had apparently caused psychological trauma and upset her so much that she had not been able to work since she had left hospital. (As far as I remember, she hadn't worked before coming into hospital.) She was also threatening to claim compensation via 'no-win, no-fee' lawyers (I doubted that they would take her case on, but she was threatening none the less).

Instead of this patient's complaint being filed under W for waste of time, my bosses had to do an investigation. My integrity was called into question, along with my patient manner – something which I am particularly proud of. A grovelling letter was sent back which I fundamentally disagreed with. Money and time were wasted. I am now constantly worried that I will get more letters and more investigations even though all I was trying to do was help her.

I completely agree that doctors should be investigated and complaints looked at if their personal or clinical skills are lacking. But I think the complaining society is spreading too far. If we worry that every bit of advice given may lead to a complaint, then doctors will act in a way to stop themselves getting in trouble and perhaps not always act in the patient's best interest.

If this 'no-win, no-fee' culture continues not only will the NHS be bankrupt from payments but it will also be bankrupt from doctors ordering too many investigations as they will treat people in a 'defensive way' (i.e. not in the patient's best interest but in a way that no one could ever complain about, as they will have carried out every possible test – even unnecessary ones). These worries pervade us as we work. Quite rightly the 'doctor knows best' culture is leaving medicine. But when we live in constant fear of litigation and worry excessively about every decision, then no wonder doctors and nurses are leaving the profession.

Why I am glad I am an A&E doctor

Today I saw a lady who was really unhappy with herself and the world. However, she made me realise why I am suited to being an A&E doctor. She was 59, depressed and had had chronic abdominal, back and head aches. She had come to A&E as she was feeling a bit worse than normal. I went to chat to her and within minutes I too became depressed and had a headache.

There was nothing really wrong with her at all. I did some blood tests to appease her and reassure myself that I wasn't missing anything. They were all normal. I told her so, and said that I didn't know what was causing her problems. I explained that she didn't need admission to hospital as there was no acute problem. All I could do was give her pain killers and get her to see her GP. I left feeling very miserable and depressed – I hadn't really helped her and both of us left feeling a bit dissatisfied.

However, I am so glad that I saw her as she made me realise what is the beautiful part of being an A&E doctor. There are so many 'heart sink' patients that we can't really sort out. They keep coming back to their GP and clinics and it is depressing for the doctor and the patient (who has often got underlying problems – though not necessarily medical ones). In my line of work, I only have to see these 'heart sink' patients once, whereas their GP has to try and work with them over and over to get to the root of their problems. I admire GPs who can deal with these patients over and over and still remain objective – I'm just glad I'm not one of them.

Not enough beds

Today, yet again, there were patients lying in A&E trolleys as there were not enough beds to go to. The hospital 'bed' manager even had to call up the local GPs requesting that they refer as few patients as possible as the hospital couldn't cope. He also came round to me and was basically pleading with me to not refer any patients for admission. What a ridiculous thing for a bed manager to be forced to do. What a wonderful NHS we have at present. I need to treat my patients in the best possible way, not with the pressure of knowing that there is a 'bed crisis' all the time.

It drives me mad when I read that the problem with the NHS is that there are too many hospital beds and that the NHS would improve if we closed beds and got patients cared for in the community. Our wards are swamped with well patients awaiting social services placement and, sadly, also awaiting a hospital-acquired pneumonia. Until adequate community care is in place, we shouldn't be closing any beds. However, at my hospital we have. A ward has been closed to save money. To house the extra patients, the medical assessment ward has become a traditional ward with one patient staying over four weeks on a supposedly short-stay emergency ward.

This means that, when A&E have stabilised the patients and referred them for hospital treatment, there is an unnecessary extended wait before they go to the ward. It has become a bit reminiscent of the A&Es of 10 years ago, with patients waiting for hours for a hospital bed. The A&E nurses have to act as ward nurses and the new patients that are arriving are given less than perfect care. It is bollocks that we need fewer beds.

Cutting bed numbers truly buggers up the quality of care that patients receive and has a damaging effect on the efficiency of the hospital. It is sad that the notification of the death of a patient on a ward is received with gratitude by the bed manager as it means that one of the A&E patients could get a bed... and I thought this was meant to be the best year ever for the NHS.

Satisfied doctor and patient

There was nothing particularly unusual today at work. It was just quite a satisfying day. No-one was particularly ill, but those that were all had readily treatable conditions. My treatments resulted in instant improvements, gratitude from the patients and satisfaction for me. They made me feel that I sometimes do useful things as opposed to practising 'defensive medicine', getting stressed by targets and doing audits showing up problems that I know will not change.

The first patient was 26 and had a dislocated shoulder. He had fallen off his skateboard. I gave him some sedation and pulled the shoulder back into place. (Sedation relaxes your muscles and also has the added benefit of making the patient amnesic so they don't remember the pain of the relocation. If you were so inclined, you could take the piss out him still skateboarding at 26, without him remembering the conversation.) When the shoulder went back in, the release of pain was enormous.

The next patient had fluid on the lungs and was really short of breath. A couple of drugs and some oxygen and within 1 hour she was a different patient. I felt quite happy.

Then a child came in with a 'pulled elbow'. It is a condition where the elbow slips from its ligaments, often when they have been 'yanked' up. They just don't use the arm. Some gentle manipulation and within 15 minutes they are back to normal.

Later in the evening we had a diabetic patient brought in unconscious by her panicking friend. A simple sugar test told us that she needed an injection of a drug to reverse the insulin she had taken without eating. Within minutes the patient was back to normal and the friend was impressed by our quick actions and calm attitude (as were the patient's parents) – and told us so.

Just before I was about to leave for home, I was asked to see a man in excruciating abdominal pain. A quick assessment and I realised that his bladder was blocked. I inserted a catheter and his pain vanished within minutes.

I drove home and thought that work is quite good fun; I am lucky I do what I do. I didn't moan once in the pub that night.

Mad bureaucracy

There are some rules in the NHS that I just don't understand. Today, I had a patient who needed blood tests. I asked one of the nurses, who wasn't busy, to take them for me and she was very happy to do so.

She was an experienced nurse, and had just got promotion to become a sister. She normally takes blood without any problems, having had the appropriate training by her last hospital trust. However, since she had moved hospitals, she apparently is not allowed to do it until she has been on a course and had 10 patients signed off. This is ridiculous. Junior doctors, who have only seen blood being taken a couple of times, are let loose to do their best as soon as they qualify. But here was an experienced nurse not being allowed to do a job she was perfectly capable of, because of bureaucracy. Let nurses' skills transfer between hospitals and let's have less form-filling and more caring.

NHS Direct... to A&E

Two patients I saw today had been told by NHS Direct to call an ambulance and come straight away. The first was a sore throat and the second a case of long-standing arthritis. They were fine and didn't need to be in A&E. I was initially annoyed, but after speaking to a friend who works at NHS Direct, my annoyance left and was replaced by pity for their difficult working environment.

I can see why the government has promoted NHS Direct. It is a great shiny thing to show off to the voters. And it is good in some respects – it is good for non-urgent advice (for example, it gave my friend fantastic advice on their non-sleeping newborn). However, for emergencies it is not so good. First of all they take a long time to get through to and second, they can't see the patient or get a general feel for how they are. Third, the treatments and advice are very protocol-driven and the staff that man the phones have got to be safe.

Hence, when there is something confusing going on, their frequent conclusion is to advise people to go to A&E... and we see some spectacularly inappropriate attendances. The sore throat clearly went down an 'airway obstruction' protocol (why else was an ambulance called?) and the hip pain must have gone down a 'fractured leg' pathway. It is not the nurse advisors' fault, they are just doing their job. People often cannot describe their symptoms clearly and when someone can't see the patient, they have to err on the side of caution. Anyway, we never hear about the ones that they prevent from coming in. Last but not least, I am sure that people lie and say NHS Direct told them to come, to lay the blame on someone other than themselves once they realise that maybe A&E is not quite where they should be.

While I think NHS Direct has its uses, I can't help but think that there may be a more efficient and safer way to help potential patients. How about more triage nurses in A&E who can give out advice? Because the patient is right in front of them they can evaluate the problem safely. Or how about taking a step back in time and paying for an out-of-hours GP service where these patients in distress would actually get a home visit at night as opposed to a protocol telling them to call an ambulance?

In the meantime, it looks as if NHS Direct is here to stay and will continue to be nicknamed NHS direct to A&E.

Why I hate laziness

I hate lazy people. Whether they work in and around A&E and delay treatment, or whether their actions force someone to come unnecessarily to A&E. All in all, laziness is not good for patient care. Last night I had three cases that really upset me.

A psychiatric patient was sent in from the local unit by ambulance. It was 3 a.m. and the nurses had called the psychiatric doctor to go and see the patient but he couldn't be bothered. The patient was short of breath so the psychiatric doctor, instead of getting off his lazy arse to assess the situation, just told him to call an ambulance. When the patient arrived, there was a very distraught family. The patient had severe dementia, and had recently developed a chest infection. Documented in the notes was a plan not to transfer the patient to hospital if she deteriorated, but let her slip away peacefully. But as no one could be bothered to properly assess the patient she was sent to the dumping ground known as A&E.

I also saw a lady with a sore throat. I explained that she didn't need to come to A&E. She told me that the GP had told her to come as he was too busy. I phoned the out-of-hours GP receptionist who confirmed that the GP was 'surfing' the net and I informed him that I was sending the patient to him. When I asked the GP why he had told this lady to come to

A&E, I was told that he was there for emergencies only. Hang on... Wasn't that my job? What a lazy (but no doubt well paid) colleague.

Then I saw a badly injured motorcyclist (otherwise known as an organ donor). His neck was painful and he needed a CT scan of the neck and head to rule out injury. The head was normal and we got a report for that (it is whizzed across to the radiologist's phone line and down their computer so they don't need to get out of bed to report it). However, to report the CT scan of the neck, the radiologist needed to come into the hospital. Instead of coming in at 1 a.m., he told us to keep the patient's neck immobilised and he would report it in the morning when he was coming in anyway. So this poor fellow had to stay strapped down all night and not move. The nurses had to log-roll him whenever he needed to vomit and I had to make up a pathetic lie of why we couldn't get the CT results straight away. Amazingly, he thought his treatment had been brilliant. It is fantastic how a few half-truths can placate most patients and hide them from the real cause of their delays and difficulties.

All I can say is that the vast majority of my colleagues are not like this. It is only a very select few. The only downside is that I only write when I am angry and so you rarely get to hear about when people have put themselves out and been helpful. But then that's life really – no-one ever praises the good guys, they just moan about the baddies. Sorry.

MRSA: the good, bad and ugly

The bad and ugly

A little known fact: one in three of us have MRSA (methicillin-resistant *Staphylococcus aureus*). It is a nasty bug that cannot be killed by the common antibiotics. Normally, it lives up your nose, getting on with its own little life and never bothering you. However, if you are vulnerable (i.e. elderly or have open wounds, etc.) it does cause problems.

A well known fact: MRSA can be transferred from patient to patient by poor hygiene and lack of proper hand washing. If you are unlucky enough to get it, then its consequences can be devastating

A little known fact: it's not *all* doctors' fault. There are things all of us need do, such as hand washing. It is also true that some doctors don't help at all, but there are other causes.

I was at work today and went to clean my hands with alcohol gel between seeing patients. I squeezed at the dispenser and nothing came out. I went to the next one and again nothing came out. It was a real effort to get anything to clean my hands with.

Later on, I went to the toilet. There was no soap, so I went to another toilet. There were no hand towels left either, so now my hands were left to dry in the air (a great way to encourage MRSA). I saw another patient and, as can often happen, I got some vomit on my clothes. I would have to take them home myself and wash somebody else's bodily fluids off in my washing machine. I don't particularly like doing that and, anyway, my machine is not specifically designed to be a sterilising washer. When I wear that top, how can I be sure it won't be harbouring any bugs?

I then saw some important-looking people – they had clipboards and ties on. I have stopped wearing a tie because of evidence that they may harbour MRSA bugs, but these men in suits didn't seem bothered. Walking through the department were some workmen. Their muddied boots left dirt all along the corridor outside the department. When the cleaners were called they acted with the speed of a very slow snail that had been smoking weed and had a heavy weight tied to its shell.

A patient with a gynaecological problem then came in. There were no clean cubicles to see her in. As she was in so much pain, there was no time to get a thorough clean of a room done before seeing her. In the corner of the room, I saw spots of dried old blood. I hope she didn't notice them.

Then I overheard a conversation between the bed manager and the ward nurse. A patient had recently died in a bed and the bed manager was trying to rush an A&E patient up to their bed. This was done despite the ward wanting a bit longer to get the area thoroughly cleaned.

Later, A&E became even busier and so we had to fit two patients into a space designed for only one. This occurs on a weekly basis. The proximity of the patients surely cannot help when it comes to trying to stop hospital-acquired infections.

After work, I went to see a friend who had just given birth earlier that day. She was at another hospital, but there were the same problems. Her mother had complained to the midwives about old blood on the floor. The answer she got was that the cleaning 'manager' had been informed. But 3 hours later, there was still no cleaner. Different hospital, same problems. At the same time, everywhere I looked – at both hospitals – there were expensive posters on the walls, advising doctors and nurses about washing our hands. From the above examples, surely managers can realise that it's not all our fault – they have to look at more fundamental causes.

These are the effects of bad management and bad politics. During the Thatcher era hospital cleaning services were privatised and given to the company that offered the lowest price as long as they promised to maintain basic standards. The cleaners working for us in A&E do a fantastic job, considering the pay and the conditions they have to work under. But they are often on temporary contracts. If you are in this situation, you may not care as much as someone on a permanent contract and with a decent wage. When the cleaning managers' priority is their shareholders and not necessarily providing as good a service as possible to the hospital, then no wonder there are occasions when I can't find hand towels and soap.

However, there is a more fundamental problem leading to high hospital-acquired infection rates. When hospitals work at 100 per cent capacity, then there is not enough time to clean properly between patients using the same bed. So when you think about MRSA, don't just blame doctors and nurses – we need a kick up the arse but so do the politicians and managers.

The good

Lots of patients are not happy when we discharge them. They feel that they need hospital admission even when this is not the case. It is often a hard argument to persuade them otherwise. It is an argument made easier when you remind them about the risks of coming into hospital: hospital-acquired infections.

Errr, I think he has vffxyeez syndrome

This is a true story that has been slightly exaggerated for artistic reasons, but is essentially what happened at work today.

I saw a 28-year-old today. A nice bloke, except for some quite ridiculous 1970s 'love' and 'hate' tattoos on his knuckles. He also had a tattoo on his chest saying 'Danielle 4 ever 2gether never 2part' entwined in a heart – I found out subsequently that they split up six months ago.

Anyway, he had appendicitis. So, I called the surgical doctor.

'...yarrr. He hazzz vycchxty.'

'Huh?', I said.

'vcdftys. Yah zloba hytchytd.'

'Um... Could you please come take his appendix out, otherwise he will get septicaemia and die.'

'Yarrrr. zeeee sabch I mean vzyxhcz.'

'... And Danielle might become a bit more sympathetic and then they might get back together.'

'Yar. meesaztre.'

'Uh... why don't you come down to A&E, it must be the phone line'

It wasn't. The phone line was BT and excellent. My communication skills were fine. So were his – if he was in Poland.

So I decided on a game of Pictionary to explain what I thought was wrong. At last we understood each other. I drew a picture of an appendix and a man crying, he smiled and raised his thumbs and 4 hours later the man was being operated on by the boss of our Polish friend. All I can say is thank God for Pictionary – an international life-saving game. It made me think: how did this obviously competent and friendly doctor, but someone who cannot speak English that well, get to work here? The answer is the European Union and stupid rules.

Now, I love Europe – from French sophistication to German efficiency, Spanish flair to the Italians' generally fantastic bums. I love the European Union – security in our continent for the last 50 years and international cooperation – and I look forward to a single currency instead of having to look at the queen's face every day (if we had to have a British queen on our money I would prefer Elton John or Brian from *Big Brother*).

I am also in agreement with most of the EU treaties, such as the common trade agreements. I also approve of the European working time directive, which has meant that I know what my kid looks like and improved the frequency of when I can see my mates (my mum-in-law still thinks I do a 90-hour week, though, and I am in no rush to tell her about the 56-hour limit). Until recently the only thing I wanted to change about Europe was to bring in a treaty banning female underarm hair.

However, things have changed... new freedom of work laws means that you have the right to work in any European Union country, without a language test. For very junior doctor jobs – F1/F2 – you don't always need an interview, although I understand (hopefully) that is changing. Also, increasing numbers of European doctors wanting to work in England has meant that there are too many doctors for too few jobs. So the government has decided that non-EU doctors who have passed English tests, who have lived in England for many years and who may have English as their first language are positively discriminated AGAINST and jobs are given to these EU doctors instead – who because of EU rules do not have to take English language tests before they work here. They may be the best doctors in the world but if they cannot converse with their patients and colleagues then they are not going to be any good.

Our government's idea of gratitude to the thousands of Asian/Australasian/South African doctors who have kept our NHS running the past 30 years, during severe doctor shortages, is to say 'Piss off. We are instead going to employ EU doctors who may or may not be able to speak English.' There isn't even a test to see if they know how to play Pictionary, for shit's sake!

The government needs to do what other EU countries do and ignore ill-thought-out laws or at least make sure that non-British doctors must be interviewed so that we know they can at least speak English – even if they are going to be doing a locum job for only a couple of days.

This is not an anti-EU rant, this is a plea for better scrutiny of our doctors. Forget about political correctness and have some common sense. The Polish doctor I was working with was an excellent and incredibly hard-working doctor. I welcome his skills, expertise and knowledge, but just wish he could speak English better before working here.

I spent the whole day fuming… until I had a Polish patient who couldn't speak English. I had to call my new Polish doctor friend back to translate… he used Pictionary with me to explain that he was a trainee surgeon and not a free translation service. So, Pictionary can be used as a life-saving tool and to express your anger. My type of game.

What's wrong with me?

I went to the pub tonight and people were worried. I wasn't myself. I have never been like this before. I was quiet and didn't moan once. I went on about how wonderful work was today. It was the first day I had used our new hospital CT scanner and the pictures it produced were a pleasure to behold. I also went on about how wonderful it is that we have an additional psychiatry liaison nurse working in A&E today. I mentioned that I had got a thank you letter and how supportive my consultants were when I was running into difficulties with a really sick patient earlier in the morning.

Later in the evening I sat next to a member of the ambulance service, who had started his first day as a new emergency care practitioner. This is a new role invented by the government where ambulance personnel go to patients' houses and try and sort them out there and then as opposed to bringing them to A&E. Apparently, in his first day at work he had prevented five A&E attendances. I told him how I thought that his new post could drastically improve care and what a fantastic use of money it was. For the first time in a long time I was not being sarcastic.

It was weird being this positive about the NHS – a very rare experience. It also meant I had a miserable time at the pub as I had nothing to moan about and ranting is my favourite hobby.

Luckily, today was a rare exception. The usual shit and problems recurred the next day and I had a happier time at the pub.

When not to get ill

I dread the beginning of August – especially the first Wednesday in August. It is when all the newly qualified doctors start. Genius medical planning supervisors have decided to make this the date when all other junior doctors rotate jobs as well – another consequence of MMC, which no one seems to have thought through. This is always a nightmare time in hospitals as frequently all the junior doctors are not only new to the hospital but also to the job. The doctors you are working with need a lot of supervision. Some of the doctors you refer to will also be new and although they may be the specialists they might not be able to give much 'specialist' help... it is something to think about when you are planning when to have your next heart attack.

Other times to avoid getting ill are the last Friday of the month. Working in a hospital is a very social affair and once a month there is a big Thursday night out – to celebrate pay day. Often the nights are organised with the other emergency services, so called 999 nights, where doctors try their luck with police ladies/men and the firemen get to try it on with nurses. Booze flows and everyone enjoys themselves... unfortunately, they have to come to work the next day.

ℒ Out-of-hours GPs

A few years ago the government went into negotiation with GPs about a new contract. Everyone agrees that the government negotiators got well and truly shafted. The GPs managed to negotiate themselves out of night work and Saturday work for a relatively small loss of wages (which could easily be made up elsewhere in the new contract). Responsibility for the patient's care was also transferred from the GP to the PCT. As anyone who has ever tried to get a GP out of hours knows, the service is not as good as it used to be. Instead of being able to see a GP who works in the practice you go to, you speak to a central triage service run by a 'cooperative' or private company and a GP triages your call. They either ask you to come to the out-of-hours GP service, often situated near your local hospital, or they go and see you at home, or they tell you to go to A&E. The problem is that the GP has no knowledge of you and does not have access to your GP notes.

The other problem is the way these cooperatives are run. There are only a few (well paid) GPs working at a time and so their time is limited. The chances of them telling you to go to A&E as opposed to doing a home visit are now inappropriately high. These GPs are mostly locums and are on an hourly rate, at a rate that is massively greater than any senior A&E doctor could ever dream of.

So if your gran has a chest infection outside 9–6, the out-of-hours GP may now advise her to go straight to A&E – there are not enough of them working to enable them to go and see everyone who needs a home visit. Previously, they would go and visit to determine whether such patients needed hospital admission. If they could cope with oral antibiotics, then they prescribed them and organised their regular GP to review them in a couple of days' time. If the patients needed hospital admission, they organised a bed and referred it directly to the medical team and directly to a hospital bed.

I had a similar experience two days ago. A 94-year-old bed-bound patient came in by ambulance from a nursing home. The carers had called the GP as she was a bit more chesty than usual. The out-of-hours GP stated that he was too busy to come and see her and that if the carers were concerned then they should call an ambulance. So an ambulance was called and I saw her. She was quite well, but the nurses were right, she had a chest infection and needed oral antibiotics. I prescribed them and gave her a week's course, but she couldn't get home as it was now after 11 p.m. and, as discussed before, we don't have a contract with the ambulance service for non-urgent transfers after hours. She had to stay the night and was distressed... and she was exposed to other patients' germs and other patients on the ward were exposed to hers. This was all because a GP would not go and see her. I don't blame the individual GP as he was probably too busy but do blame the system that has been brought into place which makes this commonplace.

The government has written a paper – *Direction of Travel for Urgent Care; a Discussion Document* – containing all these suggestions on how to prevent hospital admissions and A&E attendances. They talk about 'patient centred plans' which are to be used after hours: for example, health workers visiting people in their home to give them appropriate treatment and arranging extra help at home. What a fantastic idea! But hang on a sec... these were services that used to be provided out of hours by GPs. The government is the one who took away the out-of-hours responsibility from GPs and is now bemoaning the fact that the level of care has gone down and hospital admissions up. Politicians talk a good game but are not so good on the actions bit. I don't think at present I would trust the government to run a bath, let alone the NHS.

It is incredibly important to run out-of-hours care properly and efficiently. We need a rethink. True accidents and emergencies should come to A&E – no argument there. Elderly people who need to be seen at home should be seen by GPs (if medically unwell) and minor injuries and the like should be seen by the new breed of paramedics – emergency care practitioners, who can do things such as suture wounds, etc. The GPs' databases of notes should be freely available to these health professionals out of hours.

Anyone else should come to A&E and be seen by a triage nurse. She can determine if they are sick enough to warrant the specialist skills of an A&E doctor. If, however, someone has a minor injury, then they could be seen by an emergency care practitioner (with supervision and advice from senior A&E doctors) or, if they have a primary care problem, then they could be seen by a GP based in or near to the A&E department. Everybody would work together and there would be a parity of pay for out-of-hours work between the hospital staff and GPs.

The government would like to think that this is what its policies have tried to create via creating new 'urgent care centres', but the reality is we are a very long way from this particular Utopia.

℞ Sick outside 9–5, Monday to Friday?

Working hours are only about a quarter of the hours in the week. I have a secret that I want NHS managers to know – people get ill outside these times. This, however, doesn't mean they don't deserve the same standard of care.

From lack of access to GPs, to A&E doctors often being more junior at night and not being able to get investigations done, people don't always get optimum care if they are ill outside the hours of 9–5.

I have had several cases recently that have really upset me. For example, a 26-year-old student nurse came in at 9 p.m. on a Thursday. He had come off his mountain bike and had immediately fitted for 1 minute as a result of the head injury he sustained. This is an indication for an urgent scan. There are even guidelines produced by the National Institute of Clinical Excellence (NICE) saying that a scan is indicated. However, there is a shortage of radiologists at my hospital and they have a very harsh on-call regime. Therefore, there can be occasional resistance to moderately urgent scan requests such as this one.

I saw the patient and tried to organise a scan. The request was deemed 'non-urgent' by my seniors and the radiologist and was turned down. He had to wait until morning. If he had come in between 9 a.m. and 5 p.m., then he would have had the scan without any arguments. Luckily, it was normal, which prompted everyone to say, 'See, we told you so' and 'You didn't have to worry'. But it might not have been normal and he could have been sitting there with bleeding in his brain all night. I also had to explain to the patient why he wasn't going to have a scan immediately when I believed he needed one.

Another patient came in on the Saturday of a bank holiday weekend. She was eight weeks pregnant and had had a vaginal bleed – possibly a miscarriage. She was desperate for a child and had already had three miscarriages. She was distraught. I examined her and her abdomen was soft and pulse was normal – she did not have any worrying signs prompting an urgent scan. However, she needed one for her psychological well-being. The next 'Early Pregnancy Clinic' appointment was in three days' time. The gynaecologists at the hospital said they wouldn't do one because they were too busy and that it wasn't an appropriate 'out-of-hours' request. I felt awful for her, but there was nothing I could do but send her home with my heartfelt apologies and 'unreassuring' reassurance.

Another patient came with an attempted suicide. He was very distressed and he needed to see a psychiatrist. However, the psychiatrist was doing a 24-hour shift and was on 'protected sleep' except for dire emergencies. He could wait to see the psychiatrist on our observation ward, but this only added to his distress.

There are numerous other examples of the problems of out-of-hours care. The NHS should be planned so that you can expect the same level of care whatever time of day you are ill. People should do only a maximum of 12-hour shifts so that there is no such thing as 'protected sleep', and so we can get specialist doctors down to A&E at all hours of the night even if the patient's condition is not life threatening.

Whatever the problems are, surely A&E needs to be able to get specialist help 24 hours a day? The resources need to be made available so that this happens. Specialist help is available for life-threatening conditions 24 hours a day, 7 days a week. But perhaps it also needs to be available 24 hours a day for less important, but still potentially treatment-altering reasons, if only to speed up patient care and reduce the number of unnecessary admissions (and hence also save money). We live in a 24/7 society – surely it is time the NHS joined the twenty-first century.

A sick man

His pulse was getting weaker and weaker. Shit, I had given him too much of the sedative drug. Shit! Shit! Shit! I got an ECG. His rhythm had changed into an irregular one. I started another drug. It didn't work. He was starting to become unconscious. I tried to call out to the nurses to get the consultant in to help me, but nothing came out. I had to take over this patient's breathing. I tried to intubate him, but I just kept on getting the tube in the gullet and not the windpipe. His oxygen levels were falling. My pulse was racing. I called for an anaesthetist and finally someone came running to help. But he was dressed as Pudsey Bear. I begged my wife to help. Hang on... What the hell was my wife doing at work, holding my hand? Why was the anaesthetist dressed as Pudsey Bear? What the hell was going on? I breathed a sigh of relief. I was dreaming again. There was no sick man and I could get back to sleep, knowing that I hadn't been party to anyone's demise in the last few hours.

But there was one sick man. Me. Why can't I sleep well at night? Why do I ruminate about problems? Why do I worry so much about how I treat patients? And, what is worse, spending all my time worrying and driving my wife mad, or not worrying at all?

Why I love A&E

The wonder of A&E is that you never know what is going to happen and who or what is going to walk through the doors. It is not like being a specialist doctor, where you will only see packaged patients who fit a certain criterion. That would drive me crazy. I love the unknown.

It was 4 a.m. when the ambulance brought us an 86-year-old man from a nursing home. He was unconscious. As he arrived, I directed the ambulance into the Resus area. I grabbed my junior colleague and went through the set pattern of treating people when they are sick and you haven't got a clue what is going on. It's the ABCDE approach. Basically, you treat the things that could kill them first and then move on.

A is for airway Check the airway. This gentleman couldn't keep his airway open because he was unconscious. He was at risk of dying from a lack of oxygen. To solve this problem, I inserted a naso-pharyngeal airway – a small tube that goes through the nose to the back of the throat. It means that even if the patient is unconscious, they cannot block their windpipe with their tongue. It can appear a bit barbaric to do, and it's not particularly nice for relatives to see – but it is simple and life saving.

B is for breathing Check the breathing. He wasn't breathing well enough and so I gave him oxygen – again ridiculously easy and cheap and a life saver. You then move on to C.

C is for circulation His blood pressure was low, so we inserted a cannula and gave him intravenous fluids. This brought up his blood pressure, thereby improving his circulation. We then moved on.

D is for disability Find out how unconscious he is and then look for a cause. He was very unconscious and it soon became obvious on examination that he had had a major stroke.

E is for exposure Examine the rest of him – is anything else going on, for example hidden injuries, etc.

At this point his respiration became more and more erratic. I thought that it was because of the swelling from the stroke pressing on the brain. I thought he might 'arrest' (i.e. his heart and breathing stop). I then had to make a very quick decision as to whether trying to restart his heart would be a good idea.

There are three main questions that must be asked at times like this: first, what was his quality of life like before?; second, what are his chances of surviving the cardiac arrest and then the subsequent treatment?; and third, what are his wishes, either expressed by him or by his relatives?

There are two common misconceptions here. First, the decision whether to restart a heart is ultimately the doctors' and not the relatives'. I know some doctors make patients' relatives feel that they are making the decision – well, they are not. It leads to relatives feeling guilty and that is not fair.

Consult them and take their opinions into account. But do not let them decide.

Second, 'not for Resus' does not mean not for treatment. You can have full, active treatment to try and prevent a cardiac arrest, but not resuscitation – basically if the treatment has not stopped you having a terminal event (i.e. a cardiac arrest) then nothing we do as doctors will change that. To proceed with a resuscitation attempt under these conditions is fruitless and cruel. The same applies (and a lot of doctors don't get this one – and it is also only my opinion and not necessarily medical gospel) if your underlying condition means that any treatment in intensive care would ultimately be futile. You can survive a prolonged resuscitation only if you go to intensive care afterwards. If that is not appropriate, then what is the point in trying to stop you dying now, only to die 2 hours later but with multiple rib fractures?

I spoke to the nursing home. The patient had a poor quality of life, didn't get out of his wheelchair and had multiple medical problems. If he did arrest, his medical problems might hinder any resuscitation attempt and his quality of life was such that we might be making things worse rather than better. Therefore, he was a patient whom I indicated not for Resus (or intensive care) but for active treatment – we gave him fluids and oxygen. I called his son in.

By then I thought he was going to die. I explained to the son what had happened and what we were doing. Although we couldn't save his life, I think we made the inevitable death easier for his son to bear. We then handed over care of the patient to the medical doctors who would provide ongoing care. He died the next day with his family around him.

Patients' wrong priorities

Part of the fun of working in A&E is that you get to work with challenging patients who are accompanied by the police. A lot of doctors hate working with this subsection of the community, but I find it… interesting.

Last night I saw a patient who had strong personality traits that other people might find offensive, but which I, as a doctor, couldn't possibly comment on. He had nicked a car, then been chased by the police. He crashed at about 90 m.p.h. and was thrown about 20 metres along the ground. He tried to run away, but with one leg at a completely unnatural angle to the rest of his body; he only managed to get as far as a waiting ambulance.

The ambulance service called us up to let us know what was coming in. A trauma call was put out. When he arrived he was in a bad state. His leg was mangled, but it was important to not just focus on the obvious injury and ensure that the rest of him was not in trouble, especially his lungs, heart and abdomen. We went through the usual treatment of my colleagues assessing him while I explained to him what was happening and getting relevant information.

'How old are you, what medical problems have you got, any allergies, do you take any medications?' I asked.

His answers were not that helpful. 'Get the f**k off me and get those f**king stupid things off my neck.'

I tried to explain that those things were neck blocks, which were protecting his neck in case he had damaged his cervical vertebrae and possibly his spinal cord. I again explained what we were going to do to him – give him fluids and pain relief, take blood tests, examine him and organise some scans if necessary. He seemed a little bit quieter for 10 seconds, but then he started again.

'Who the f**k is cutting my f**king T-shirt? That cost a thousand pounds. I am going to sue you, you bastard.'

The nurse apologised and explained why she had cut it – so that I could examine his chest easily – and said we had spares he could have afterwards. He thanked her by spitting in her face and accusing her of being a lady of loose morals. For A&E doctors at this stage, it can be very difficult. Is the patient acting this way because this is their normal behaviour pattern – or are they acting in that way due to pain, fright, lack of oxygen and/or brain damage? And if you treat them against their will, are you doing it in their best interest because they are not in a rational state or are you assaulting them? These are all judgment calls, with no right or wrong answers, which makes A&E doctors' and nurses' jobs interesting but frequently difficult.

All his observations were so far normal, and he had no obvious head injury of note. I therefore decided that he was acting in this manner because he wasn't the most pleasant of people. He started to swear about the neck brace and collar again.

'Look mate. We are cutting off your T-shirt because we want to examine your chest and I do not think the T-shirt cost a grand – even if it is a real Ralph Lauren one. As for your neck brace, we will take it off as soon as we have X-rayed your neck.'

He didn't seem satisfied.

'F**k the lot of you. I am out of here.'

He ripped the collar off, put the nurses at risk by pulling out his cannula and somehow stormed as far as the end of the resuscitation room, where he was nicked for stealing cars and dangerous driving. This was quite a feat with a broken leg, but it is amazing what the power of the mind and the thought of being nicked (oh, and a temporary plaster cast) will do. After he realised his fate, he accepted treatment and was in theatre later that night to have his leg fixed properly.

How to be seen quickly

Ever gone to A&E and been frustrated at having to wait 3 hours and 59 minutes to be seen and sorted out? Over the years, I have observed various methods of how to get seen quickly. Some of these methods are very inappropriate and have been used by some quite naughty patients to speed up their care at the expense of more needy patients. Please remember that by lying about symptoms, you are putting your and other people's health at risk. Don't do it please.

1. Have a genuine emergency. Best is probably your heart stopping. The ambulance will call us to tell you are coming in and you will be seen straight away. During the day, you may even see a consultant, unless they are doing something that management have deemed more urgent, such as responding to a complaint letter, filling in a compensation form or going to a meeting with a silly title such as 'Introducing a Patient Centred Care Flow Pathway: Interim Discussions'.

2. Similarly, have a serious trauma and you will have a team of doctors waiting to see you on arrival.

3. Be a child and cry a lot. If that doesn't work, cry loudly, then start to scream.

4. If you are pregnant, say you think you are having your baby. This scares A&E staff shitless and we get you a swift transfer to the maternity unit.

5. Say you have chest pain as soon as you book in with reception. Clutch your chest and say you feel sick and the pain is going down your left arm. This guarantees going to the front of the queue. Only do this if it is true. About a year ago, I had a bloke who said all this to the receptionist. I was called away from the patient I was seeing and went to see him. The pain had gone (it had never been there) and he had injured his foot playing rugby. He admitted to making it up, as he had a date that night and didn't want to be stuck in A&E.

6. If you have a minor injury, make it a really simple one such as a broken wrist that emergency nurse practitioners can treat. You don't want to have to wait to have to see a doctor.

7. Have a condition that an A&E doctor can treat and doesn't have to get specialists to see you. It is bad enough having to wait to see us, but if you have two waits then that is doubly bad. You may even get admitted to a ward unnecessarily, just so that you don't breach the government's 4-hour target.

8. Be a doctor or nurse at the hospital where you go. Or be a friend or relative of theirs and take them with you to A&E.

9. If you are a policeman, fireman or ambulance man, come in wearing your uniform so that the triage nurse knows you are 999. There are some very minor perks to serving the public.

10. Come in with police. It is not that we want to see you that quickly, but we know that the police are needed back on the streets and they don't want to be here.

11. Please note that calling an ambulance will not speed up how quickly you get seen.

12. ...Neither will saying 'NHS Direct told me to come straight away.'

13. ...Neither will saying, 'My father is a big contributor to the local area and paid for your new scanner, you know. I want to be seen now.'

14. The best one I have found, which never fails to work, is simple. Be a politician or an important hospital manager. Not only will you be seen straight away, but you will be seen by a consultant. As well as being seen straight away, you will get immediate access to any form of investigation and if you need to see a specialist, then this will happen immediately. No wonder the politicians and managers don't really know what is happening in emergency care. *Please note that this is only my prejudiced opinion and sarcastic sense of humour and not really NHS policy.*

ℒ The dangers of cannabis

It was 4 p.m. on a Thursday. I picked up the next card out of the box – a 19-year-old with personal problems, who was accompanied by his mother. No. No. No! Not another attempted suicide. It drives me mad. With people who have suicidal ideation, my sole job is to check they are medically OK and then determine if they are very suicidal and need to see the psychiatrist today or if it can wait for a GP review in a few days' time. I looked around to see if anyone would notice if I put the card back and picked up something less soul-destroying. No luck.

'What are you seeing next?' asked my consultant.

'Nineteen-year-old. Personal problem.'

'Easy,' he said. 'Just determine if they need to see a psychiatrist today or their GP in a few days time'.

'Thanks for the advice,' I said sarcastically.

'It's a bit boring, though. I'm about to see a bloke with something where it shouldn't be,' he retorted and laughed in a quite inappropriate way.

I had no idea what he was on but I smiled and answered something about how I thought psychiatry patients got a raw deal and how I was quite interested in them. It was one of those comments that you couldn't tell if you meant it sarcastically or not.

I went to the private interview room nicknamed WD40 (it is called the 'Want to Die' room and the hinges need some oil, hence the name). There I saw this very posh-looking mother and her son, who also looked very posh, except that he had an eyebrow ring, dreadlocks and was playing with a packet of Rizlas. (He was a true Trustafarian – attempting to be a hippie, but with Daddy's trust fund to support him.)

'So what's the matter?' I asked.

'What are those?' He pointed at a smoke detector. 'Turn them off; I don't want people to know what is going on.'

'They are smoke detectors. Don't worry. What's the matter?'

'Who are you?' he asked without making eye contact.

'I'm a doctor.' I turned to his mother. 'Did you bring him here?' I asked.

'Yar. I just don't know what is going on. He is not himself. He is normally so polite and nice. All he does is scream and say they are after him. I do not know who *they* are.'

'There is a battle of good and evil and they need me dead,' he interjected. 'She doesn't understand.'

The conversation continued in a similar vein and it became quite obvious that this was a not a case of suicidal ideation, but an acute psychotic paranoia episode. Not only would he need a psychiatrist to review him, but he would probably need to be admitted to a psychiatric hospital.

As I continued my questioning, it transpired that he had recently been using cannabis. It had started a year ago at his boarding school. He was destined for four As at A-level – and probably a place at Oxbridge that our class system had predetermined for him – but he started to smoke dope and lost interest in most things except weed. He passed his A levels but only just. He and his parents had planned for him to go on a gap year travelling to find himself and the true meaning to life, or study pottery at St Martin's College of Art or something like that.He never found himself. All he found was a harder dealer. Over the last few weeks he had been buying skunk – stronger cannabis than what he was used to. That was when the paranoia started. He slowly changed from a fast-food ordering, ambivalent and stoned teenager into a psychotically paranoid man.

As it was within working hours, it wasn't a fight to get a psychiatrist. Psychosis is the interesting part of psychiatry. Most of their work in A&E is now personality disorders and attempted suicides/cries for help/attention-seeking behaviour. This was good old proper psychosis, but with a new cause – very strong cannabis.

I cannot be 100 per cent sure that this lad was psychotic because of the cannabis. However, there is a correlation between cannabis use and psychosis and schizophrenia. Whether it is a cause or a correlation, no-one can be sure, but both are on the rise in society and so I reckon that cannabis is at least a causative factor.

So, despite the evidence of this, the government confused the law and people thought that cannabis had been decriminalised. What folly. People like this lad were not scared of the consequences of taking this very strong hallucinogenic drug and so built up an addiction. So what's my solution? I think the answer is legalising the drug. These two facts are not contradictory. Let me explain.

Cannabis use is widespread in teenagers and the young adult population – 40 per cent of people under 20 have taken it. When I was a teenager, the cannabis on the street was relatively mild but now the dealers are selling stronger and stronger stuff.

There are two options. One is keep it illegal and punish people more severely for using it. However, that is never going to work – you can't arrest 40 per cent of the population. Prohibition doesn't work. Anyway, in some cases the police don't actively encourage it, but do turn a blind eye. For example, during the last World Cup the foreign police didn't seem to mind our football fans smoking it, as it calmed them down and stopped them beating the shit out of the opposing supporters. Medically it is, I believe, much safer to go on a one-night bender getting stoned rather than a drinking binge. I would also feel much safer walking past a group of stoned teenagers than a group of drunken ones.

The alternative is to legalise it. Then you do two things. You can control the quality and power of the drug – the weaker stuff still has the same instant relaxing effect people use it for, but is probably less likely to cause the longer term decline in function and psychosis. You then create very high sentences for dealing with other stronger forms of cannabis.

Users then have a standardised and controlled drug, which is cheaper than the dealers can sell it for and also much safer. Market forces reduce the number of dealers; fewer people go to them and so fewer people are introduced to more dangerous drugs. The cannabis can be taxed and the money spent on treating those that are addicted to drugs, while the rest of the population can make a judgment call about whether they take the drug, knowing the risks and benefits (as we all do when drinking alcohol).

Unfortunately, the government's half-way house is the worst of both worlds and is a ridiculous compromise. It has encouraged the rise of dealers selling very strong and dangerous cannabis. Please reverse this decision, and go back to the drawing board. Get a Royal Commission on how to deal with cannabis and generally tackle drugs in society – but please get some A&E doctors' advice because we deal with it and its consequences every day.

For fit's sake

There are two explanations for the events of last night. First, the organiser of the event was a complete idiot or, second, he was just sick and twisted. I hope the latter, but rather think it's the former. Imagine you were in charge of an Alcoholics Anonymous summer party. Would you take them drinking? No! Or a vegetarian community group, would you take them to a slaughter house? No! Or a nudist group, would you take them clothes shopping? No... but why not? Because it would probably upset them and make them ill.

So why on earth did a local epileptic support group on a summer weekend away organise a disco with strobe lighting? You couldn't make it up. It was epilepsy city in my A&E. Two fitters, one pseudo fitter – he made it up 'cos he was feeling left out. (You can tell if a fitter is making it up by dropping their arm on their face: if it hits the face, they are not making it up but if they move the arm so that it doesn't hit them, then they are making it up.) Two people also attended A&E because they thought they might have a fit, one carer came with chest pain and one with stress. Luckily, it wasn't too busy an evening otherwise, so I saw the funny side.

The best bit came when a druggie was in and saw these two people fitting, and when they woke up, asked where they got their E from as they were really moving with the beat!

℞ The state of some nursing homes

Today I had a 78-year-old confused and scared lady come in from a residential home. The ambulance form said she came in because she was short of breath. The home didn't send anyone with her and there was no accompanying letter. I phoned the home and there had been a change of shift since she had been admitted. No-one really knew what had happened or why she was sent in. I then asked for some details about her past medical history. No-one seemed to know much about that either.

This is a problem that is becoming far too frequent. It is a sad indictment of how we care for our elderly population, where homes are often run for profit and not necessarily to provide as good a service as possible. As always, when there is a problem, it gets dumped on A&E and the ambulance service. I couldn't find any new problems with her and ended up sending her back home with no change in her medications.

Why aren't GPs called out more often for these types of problems? They know their patients and know what is normal for them. Why can't homes give us a clue to the problem and send a letter or carer? Why does this happen so often? Why isn't there a word in the English language to describe me gripping my fingers and making angry facial expressions, which I could use to describe my frustrations?

℞ The best year for the NHS?

I read with interest that Patricia Hewitt, Secretary of State for Health, claimed that 2006 was the best year ever for the NHS. I really think she has lost her last marble. Yes, money has been poured in to the NHS, but in such a bad way that it has antagonised the NHS workers. For those of us who love the concept of the NHS, it has been one of the most miserable of years, not the best ever.

In 2006 we have seen plans for haphazard reorganisation lead to hospital closures without alternative options being in place. We have seen various trusts go virtually bankrupt and having to call in ridiculously expensive management consultants. There has been a loss of nursing and vital ancillary staff jobs and some trusts have seen posts for doctors frozen to save money. Meanwhile, the benefits of being an NHS hospital doctor have been eroded (e.g. by plans to reduce study budgets).

Some private finance companies are making a fortune from poorly negotiated PFI (private finance initiative) contracts and Private Treatment Centres are milking in the profits from guaranteed payments for operations that may or may not happen. The waste drives hospital doctors mad. Meanwhile, in GP land, despite their pay increases, doctors are feeling less and less motivated and more disillusioned with a centrally directed NHS and erosion of their autonomy.

However, it is not just me who believes that 2006 has been a disaster for the NHS. As the BMA (British Medical Association) council chair James Johnson said, 'Health workers and patients are paying the price for ill-thought-out government policies such as PFI and for poor NHS management that has led to job cuts and clinic closures...' (for more information see http://www.bma.org.uk/ap.nsf/Content/pr141206).

Fortunately, it is not just doctors and nurses who realise that the fundamentals of the NHS are being eroded. The campaign to keep the NHS public has seen phenomenal growth this year and the number of petitions and demonstrations about ill-planned closures has increased dramatically.

What is really amazing is that it is not just me that disagrees with the NHS reform plans as they are at present. At a hospital close to my heart, there was Hazel Blears, the chairman of the Labour Party, campaigning against the effects of her party's policies – in this case the closure of the maternity unit in Salford. Reading on the BBC website, I also learned that in April John Reid (a senior Labour politician) campaigned against closures at his local hospital (for further information see http://news.bbc.co.uk/1/hi/uk_politics/6213445.stm).

But, Mrs Blears and co. – stop being so hypocritical and NIMBYish. If you don't support these hospital closure programmes you have only got yourselves to blame. It is the effect of sofa-style government without proper scrutiny that leads to the effects of the unintended consequences. So, Blears and co., since you obviously agree with me that that these NHS reforms (which are needed) have been very badly organised and damaged the NHS, then surely you must resign from your positions and campaign for a properly run NHS. If you did this, then I would imagine that Nye Bevan might be turning that bit less in his grave.

Hoping that the ground will swallow you up

It is an easy mistake to make. You are seeing lots of patients, all of whom are new to you, and sometimes you make an assumption about a patient and the person with them. When this is wrong, it can be very embarrassing. Some of the assumptions I have made, have made me want the earth to swallow me up:

Me: ' ...And you are his mother.'
Patient's relative: 'Wife. Not mother'.
Me: 'Ah, yes. Oops'.

To a patient and relative holding hands: 'And you are her partner?'.
Relative: 'No. Brother.'

To a male relative who was there with his unconscious partner in a blond wig: 'So what happened to her tonight?'
The friend replies: 'He has been drinking. He is pre-op, darling. Pre-op. "She" is still a he. Read the name on the card. Stephen is hardly a female name is it?'.

The list goes on and on. However, I also find that some people automatically go out of their way to tell me their significance to each other.

To an elderly lady accompanying her friend: 'And you are her friend?'

'No, we are lesbian partners. We have been together now 45 years. We first met when I was only 25 and then we bought our first house together in Stockton-on-Tees. Her family never approved, but mine didn't really understand what lesbians were so just accepted that we were friends. But we are not. We are, but first and foremost we are a couple. A lesbian couple. And don't get embarrassed, it is beautiful.'

I wasn't embarrassed. I was just a little bored with the life story and felt as if I was on the set of *Little Britain*.

One of the things I tried after a spate of faux pas was to not ask what the relationship of the friend/relative is. After one experience I will not make that mistake again. There I was, asking this lady of 65 all about her abdominal problems and her regularity down below, etc., and then I said, 'I need to examine your abdomen. Would you like it if your friend was here or would you prefer me to ask him to leave?' As I said this, I looked at the slightly dishevelled man who had been standing inside the curtains throughout the whole of our consultation and who had even said 'hello' as I walked in.

'I don't really mind. But he is nothing to do with me. I thought he was with you.'

'Oh', I replied as I could hear nurses looking for the elderly patient who had been brought in for new onset confusion and had gone missing... behind my curtains.

As my experience has grown, I have decided that the easiest way is either to flatter every relative (e.g. say to a mum with her child, 'And are you her big sister?') or just put my hand out to a relative and say, 'And you are... ?' and wait for them to reply. I just wish they taught us simple tactics like that at medical school so I wouldn't have had to be so embarrassed over the last few years.

Two similar patients, but two different outcomes

You may think that wherever and whenever you go to A&E, you will get a similar standard of treatment. This is far from the truth. As well as medical expertise, it is the process of how emergency patients are cared for that really affects their outcome. I was at a recent training day when two cases were discussed that really showed this to be true.

The first was a 65-year-old man with severe pneumonia. The junior A&E doctor saw him after a wait of a couple of hours. After various tests, she had noticed how unwell he was and discussed it with her senior A&E colleague. The senior doctor advised that this patient needed a central line, and should then be transferred to ICU. Despite this, protocol in his hospital dictated that the patient be referred to the medical team first and they would have to arrange ICU admission. The senior A&E doctor couldn't sort the patient out as there was a very long wait of minors patients to see.

The man was admitted to the medical admissions unit after 3 hours and 49 minutes in A&E. After another 90-minute wait, he then saw one of the medical doctors. At this point the patient was deteriorating rapidly. His breathing was getting worse and his blood pressure was falling. The junior medical doctor was only in his second year of training as a GP. Having no experience as an emergency physician, he did not have the same grasp of the urgency of the problem as the senior A & E doctor did. They didn't see the problem of spending a long time asking detailed questions about past medical history instead of getting on and treating the life-threatening condition.

After another hour, the medical registrar came to review. He soon realised that the patient was very sick and needed this central line. However, he didn't feel confident in putting one in as it wasn't part of his routine work – he was training to be a rheumatologist and had just had a year out to do research. He asked the anaesthetist to do it for him.

After another 30-minute wait the anaesthetist came and put in the central line and treatment was started, as well as closer monitoring of his vital signs. At the same time the medical doctor referred him to ICU. The ICU doctor came down and accepted him immediately to ICU. However, they had not been prewarned to expect this patient, so spent 2 hours discharging another patient from the ICU to the ward to create a free bed. Finally, some considerable time after first coming into A&E, the patient went to ICU, where proper treatment started. However, by this time his kidneys had stopped working and he needed dialysis until he was well again. His breathing had got even worse and he had to be intubated. After a two-week stay in ICU, he died from multi-organ failure induced by the chest infection.

In this case, no individual did anything wrong, but the system was at fault, in not allowing the patient to get speedy ICU treatment. As a whole, the care was not perfect and possibly contributed to his death. As a government statistic it was great – he was seen and admitted within 4 hours of arrival in A&E. There are no stars for the quality of his care.

The second case was very similar and happened at a hospital 50 miles away from the first one (and it wasn't a centralised teaching hospital, but a bog-standard district general – the type the government don't seem to like). The difference was that they had better processes in place and had invested money in emergency nurse practitioners (ENPs).

A sick man, 68, was brought in with a very nasty chest infection. The A&E senior specialist doctor in this hospital was not busy seeing minor patients, as that was the ENP's job, and so was free to see the patient with her junior colleague. She realised immediately how sick he was.

Also, in this hospital there are very close links between ICU and A&E, which were not there in the first hospital. When the A&E doctor called, the ICU doctor took down all the information and got the unit ready to accept the patient. The unit didn't insist that the patient be seen by a medical doctor (who, remember, may not have a specialisation in acute/emergency care) but just wanted the name of the medical consultant on that day so that when the patient left ICU they had a set of doctors they could liaise with.

The A&E doctor (who is experienced in putting in central lines) inserted one into this patient while they were in the safe environment of the resuscitation room. She taught her junior doctor how to do it and so he also got training while at work. She started fluids and antibiotics. She also set up the equipment needed to monitor this man's blood pressure beat-to-beat, so they could tell exactly how he was doing. A catheter was inserted and the urine output monitored. Very soon the patient improved. After 4 hours and 30 minutes, the patient made his way up to ICU with the proper treatment well under way. He did very well and was discharged back to the ward after five days. He was home after 12 days.

While all that was happening, the ENPs were seeing the minor patients and the medical doctors were looking after their sick patients on the ward without having to be bothered by the acutely sick patient, who was being well-managed by the A&E doctor. In this case, the patient did very well but since he was in A&E for more than 4 hours the case was probably not regarded as a success in terms of targets, but was placed in the exceptions to the 4-hour rule category. There are no stars for quality of care.

Unfortunately, the process of care that the first patient got is far more common. If the money was put into acute care and the processes of delivery of care were changed, so that they were all like the second example, it would cost a bit at the beginning, but in the end would save a fortune.

One of the main reasons that these situations are so common is that the doctors working in A&E are often not experienced enough and have not had the right training to decide if the patient needs to go to ICU with the result that they are referred to the medical team. The senior doctors, who are capable of making those decisions, are often too busy trying to stop more minor cases breaching their 4-hour rule. This is a crazy situation. We should work closely with the medical doctors and make it a rule that the sickest patients should be seen by the most senior people straight away – A&E physicians or acute physicians, whoever is available at the time (it doesn't matter, as long as we are all working together).

As an aside, to get improved health care, we don't necessarily need centralised care and we certainly don't need your local district general hospital to close. There is nothing high tech about the treatment the second patient received; it was just more efficiently delivered and thus that patient had a better outcome. As my gran used to say, 'A stitch in time saves nine'; she could teach our managers a thing or two, I reckon.

An amusing patient

I couldn't swap my job for any other. Sometimes I just love being at work – especially so when you can have pleasant and amusing patients. Today I had one such patient.

Six-foot-five, built like a brick shithouse and tattoos a-plenty. When he came in he was all smiles and jokes. He had an infection at the end of his finger. He had been to his GP, who had given him antibiotics, but they hadn't worked. The pus needed to come out.

'I am afraid that I will have to make a small incision and get the pus out.'

He started to laugh, 'I am the biggest wimp in the world. Please no! I can't stand needles; I'd rather lose my finger,' he pleaded.

I told him that he very well might lose his finger and again offered him the option of an 'incision and drainage' of the abscess. He pondered, thought about a life with a nose full of bogies and opted to be brave.

I had just started to inject a tiny bit of local anaesthetic into the finger when the screaming started. Oh my God! I had never heard anything like it. But he was so embarrassed and apologetic and so nice about it, I didn't mind. I got the emergency supply of gas and air.

For simple procedures like this, gas and air (laughing gas) is hardly needed. But he needed it and boy did it work. What the gas does is to provide a small level of anaesthetic with a large amount of hysteria. You can still feel the pain, but it is no longer upsetting. You can also get the giggles. If the patient gets the giggles, then the drug is working. As long as they stay still, you can perform your operation to your heart's content. But as we all know, the giggles can become infectious. Unfortunately, once they get the giggles, then so may you. That's when the fun/difficulties start.

But you need to start the ball rolling. I started with my favourite joke for wimpish men who are having a procedure done on their arm.

I started, 'Did you hear about the patient who went to the doctor with pains in his arm? "Do you want the good news or the bad news?" the doctor inquired.

"The bad news please," said the patient.

"Well, I am afraid that we are going to have to amputate your arm."

"And the good news?" enquired the poor patient.

"The bloke in bed two wants to buy your gloves." '

Well, that got him started. The nurses groaned as they had heard it many times before. He was giggling a little at this point, but still thinking about his finger. 'Breathe more of the gas,' I said.

I went through my memory bank of shit doctor jokes. Luckily, I know a lot of them.

A patient went to his GP, 'Doctor, I don't know what the matter with me is, but I can't stop singing in a sexy Welsh accent.'

'Ah' said the doctor, 'You have Tom Jones syndrome.'

'Tom Jones syndrome?' said the patient. 'Is that common?'

The doctor responded with a little sexy dance and sang 'It's not unusual…'

The jokes were coming thick and fast. I was starting to win. The room was filling with laughter. I went for the kill. The classic man with pain everywhere he touches – he has a broken finger; the old man who has a bit of lettuce in his ear, who the doctor wants to investigate as he thinks it's a sign of something serious – the tip of the iceberg. Then my favourite: the bloke who goes to the doctor and the doctor says, 'I am afraid to tell you that you have got cancer and Alzheimer's.' 'Oh well,' the patient says. 'It could be worse – I could have cancer.'

He was in fits and it was perfect timing; with one more whoosh of the gas and air, the scalpel went in and pus upon pus upon pus came out… it was like a teenager's dream. A bandage and some antibiotics and he was on his way… all of us contented.

Closing your A&E, are they?

I work in an A&E department that the government is thinking about closing – it adds to the stress of working. The government thinks that we don't need so many A&Es and district general hospitals. It says this because:

1. Fewer people should attend A&E.
2. Most attendances are things GPs/community nurses could cope with.
3. Many conditions need home care and not hospital admission.
4. With reductions in doctors' hours, we can't have so many hospitals
5. Centralised care is better for the sickest 1–2 per cent, so sod the rest of you.

I am going to try and persuade you (just in case you needed it) why closing your local A&Es isn't such a good idea. At the same time I am going to explain why many of the problems A&Es are facing are partly caused by policies carried out by New Labour and the Tories before them.

Attendances at A&E departments are on the rise – both appropriate attendance and the inappropriate stuff we see that is neither an accident nor emergency. The fact is that people do attend… and they need treatment or reassurance or whatever. There are a number of reasons why there are increasing demands on our service. These include:

1. Alcohol – as a nation, we are getting pissed more and coming to A&E with the problems.
2. Drugs – the nation is getting higher, and when people fall they present to A&E.
3. Increasing violence in society – often resulting from factors (1) and (2).
4. Obesity – only since Jamie Oliver kicked up a fuss has Labour started doing something about it. We see

more and more obese patients with the complications that ensue.

5. Privatisation of social care – some care homes are there to make a profit and so might not always have the patient's best interests at heart. If a patient becomes a little tricky to look after, they are sometimes sent to hospital. The same goes for the privatisation of home care.

6. Encouraging (or at least not dissuading) the blame culture – the number of patients who come in because their 'no-win, no-fee,' no self-respect lawyer has told them to do so is excessive.

7. Lack of responsibility-taking – for example, I now see kids that have had a fall at school. A few years ago the school first-aider would have dealt with the scraped knee, now they are too afraid that the parents will complain.

8. The ageing society – even I can't blame that on New Labour.

There is also the problem of patients attending with GP-type problems. Yes, they should go to their GP and let me concentrate on treating the sicker patients but it is not always as simple as that. So why do they come to A&E more nowadays?

1. Loss of good-quality out-of-hours GP provision.

2. NHS Direct – it costs a lot of money and gives good advice, but at the end of the day cannot physically see patients and so takes a low-risk approach, which often means saying, 'Go to A&E'.

3. Patient choice has been encouraged – many patients now come with primary care problems, as they seem to think they can choose to come to us instead of their GP.

4. The massive influx of eastern European workers – there seems to have been no active plans to encourage them to register with GPs and so they come to A&E with their minor ailments.

With more and more people using A&E as their first point of call for many medical non-urgent problems, is it the right time to talk about closing down A&Es, without having organised the infrastructure of local community-based care? I think not.

Many conditions could be treated at home. However, we have to admit patients because support structures are not available – especially if we are trying to organise them out of 'working hours'. Admission to hospital is then the safest option. So, until a proper system of community care is sorted out, it is dangerous and unfair to local populations to close the local hospital. The other factor I think the government has forgotten, is that these patients still need to come to A&E when they are acutely ill to have their diagnosis made and then to be risk-stratified before being sent home for community care. We need a local A&E, staffed 24 hours a day for this to happen.

The government also argues that it needs to shut A&Es and local hospitals to comply with the European Working Time Directive and doctor training requirements. However, there are lots more medical students than there used to be – they will need jobs and will be happy to do shift work when they qualify. Also, all doctors are meant to have generic skills and so can cross cover. Very rarely do you need a senior orthopaedic doctor/ENT/ophthalmologist, etc., in the hospital after midnight... and if you do, then call in the consultant if you are worried. Whatever is done, it should not be used as an excuse to close hospitals, but as another reason to make junior doctors' time more efficient and relevant to training requirements.

Finally, the government's main argument is that centralising care for the most serious of cases is a good idea. I completely agree. Heart attacks and major trauma would do better in large centres where there is expertise and experience. The ambulance could take these patients directly to the most appropriate place. Consultants could work in regional teams rotating around the major centre and so those working at smaller A&E, would not become deskilled. For it to work, we would need to overcome the problem of how we are going to look after these sick patients on their long journey to regional centres, especially when our roads are so clogged up... and, remember, traffic jams are often worse when the roads have had an accident on it. The government hasn't yet got the answers in place. It seems to me that it needs a massive increase in funding for the infrastructure of pre-hospital medicine, such as having specialist doctors in ambulances and using more helicopters, before thinking about closing hospitals.

The other thing to remember is that centralising care should only affect the outcome of the sickest 1–2 per cent. So what about the other 99 per cent of patients? Centralising their care will not improve their outcome. The government should not use the centralising argument as an excuse to close local A&Es and district general hospitals (DGHs).

If anything, it will harm the health of the nation. Patients will put off travelling miles and miles to get treatment, so will get worse until they are compelled to call an ambulance. It would also be cruel to send elderly people miles and miles for non-life-threatening medical conditions such as pneumonia. The same argument goes for surgical procedures which don't need to be done at specialist centres – for example, mending broken hips. Saying that ambulances should take heart attack victims to regional centres is NOT an argument for closing your local DGH.

What really pisses me off is that Blair made a recent speech saying that he is upset that doctors are not on the streets campaigning for his reforms to be brought in more quickly. Mr Blair, I am not on the streets demonstrating because they are ill thought out and community services are not ready to take over the role of DGHs. Your successor needs to go back to the drawing board. Although your reforms *may* benefit the sickest of patients, it will not be beneficial to the other 99 per cent of patients.

Also, why didn't you tell us about it before the last election?

So, sign that petition and write to your MP. Pray that our new Prime Minister changes Blair's plans. Go on the streets and campaign to keep your local hospital A&E department. But just understand why it may be good for the ambulance to take you a bit further afield when you are having a heart attack.

Nasty walls

Many people think that there are a lot of nasty people in my town and that is why there are so many people who turn up with hand injuries from punching. I believe not. In my town, we have some really nasty walls. These walls piss people off, antagonise the good young men, shag their birds and probably their mums, and generally create trouble. That's why these walls get punched and that's why these walls need to be stopped.

I hereby pledge to campaign for the Home Secretary to introduce a wall ASBO. Lock up these evil collections of bricks which so upset these fine examples of upstanding members of the community. Make their parent ceilings pay for the damage they do to the 5th metacarpal (little finger knuckle) bone of these young upstanding members of the community. WALLS MUST BE STOPPED! WE MUST BAN WALLS FROM CITY CENTRES. This is especially so on a Friday and Saturday night when walls become especially antagonistic.

If this ban came into force, then we could virtually eradicate the broken hand problem and its victims would have no reason to come to see me at 4 a.m. It has been getting worse – yesterday I saw evidence of a wall that had teeth. This shows how nasty the walls have become.

On a serious note, if you have given someone a good punching, don't say you punched a wall. The truth is obvious and we like to know all the details... and it makes my job more interesting. If you do say that you have punched a wall, beware. You may face a sarcastic response from the doctor treating you. For example:

Dr says: 'Did the wall have teeth?'
Dr thinks: 'Tell me the truth so I know whether you need antibiotics or not.'

Dr says: 'This will hurt a little.'
Dr thinks: 'Stitching up your cut with only homoeopathic levels of local anesthetic will hopefully teach you a lesson.'

Dr says: 'You'll still have to wait for another 3 hours until I see your hand.'
Dr thinks: 'Please self-discharge.'

Dr says: 'When I get angry I say oh fiddle-dee-sticks and count to 10. Have you ever thought of that as a way of controlling your anger?'
Dr thinks: 'There are two very hard coppers with us, and you are nicked and I can joke as much as I want.'

This is just a brief synopsis of a ridiculously common injury. Let's get this wall ASBO campaign up and running. Please write to Dr Nick Edwards c/o The Friday Project.

P.S. On a serious note, even if you have got into a fight and then lied, you will still get properly treated in a non-judgmental way. The doctor just might smirk a bit behind your back. Also, if you have genuinely punched a wall then I apologise.

ℒ Tired again

It was 5 a.m. on night six of seven consecutive 12-hour shifts and I was exhausted. The last patient came in with heart failure. I examined and treated her, but her condition was nothing to get an adrenaline rush for. I think that I treated her well, but on reflection I am not sure. Did I give the right dose of morphine and frusemide? Did she really need that GTN infusion? Would I have treated her the same way if I had not been exhausted? If not, would it have been my fault?

Well, in this case I think I did do the right thing – she improved and was well enough to leave the resuscitation room and go to the ward within one and a half hours. However, I feel that there are loads of other patients that I have treated at this time of night when I may not have treated this well because I have been so tired.

Anyway, 8 a.m. came and I left for my drive home, luckily only 20 minutes away. I don't know how, but despite two strong coffees before leaving, I was driving on the main road home and then suddenly I wasn't. As the road was curling left I was sleeping. I had crossed the hard shoulder and hit the grass hill on the other side. Luckily, no-one else was involved. However, the car was destroyed, the air bags were brilliant and the police very sympathetic. An embarrassing trip back by ambulance to work, for my neck to be checked out, ensued. I was furious with myself. But again, was it all my fault or were the people who designed my rota (medical staffing) partly to blame?

While waiting for my X-ray I started to think – we are told by managers all about patient safety and how to stop causing harm to our patients. It feels (even in this no-blame culture) that doctors and nurses are taking all the blame, but the managers who design our rotas are escaping scot-free. Do airlines let their pilots work seven consecutive nights? No, it is dangerous. Are train drivers protected? Yes. Lorry drivers have maximum times they can drive for. Why? To protect you, the public. The police, ambulance and fireman – as far as I know – have had research done into night working and know that it is dangerous to do so many consecutive nights. They only do a maximum of three or four at a time. Again, safer for them and safer for the public. But doctors... sod them – let them do seven consecutive nights and let's just hope they don't kill anyone at work or on a drive home. Anyway, if they do kill someone, we can blame the doctor – we can say it is because they haven't taken part in a patient safety course, or been keen enough on continuing professional development. We can refer them to the GMC, smash their confidence and wash our hands and just say, 'Oh well, it shows that the problems in the NHS are all caused by useless doctors.'

But seriously, it is not right – it is dangerous and it does affect you. I wouldn't want to be seen by a colleague who had just done six straight nights. In the days when I first qualified, specialist junior doctors (i.e. not ones who worked in A&E – but to whom A&E referred to for admission and advice) often did 24-hour and 48-hour shifts. That was wrong but at least you got a bed and then were not on call for a few days after that. You never had to do seven consecutive nights.

The government rightly changed it, but delayed the implementation of the full working time directive and made (sorry... allowed) doctors to opt out of it. This allowed managers to devise the most dangerous working patterns – who cares if it damaged doctors and patients? What makes matters worse is that junior doctors often rotate around hospitals on training schemes. We often live 1–2 hours away, and often not near public transport. There also used to be rooms where specialist junior doctors could sleep when it wasn't busy (this was even more important for them since, unlike A&E doctors who can go home after their 12-hour shift, they often had to stay longer on the ward round telling the consultant about the patients admitted overnight). Admittedly the beds were used only occasionally – but a half-hour nap really can refresh. Now they have generally been taken away and in most cases turned into vital managers' officers – the room once referred to as 'Medical SHO On-Call Room' is now often called 'Patient Liaison Facilitator Deputy Manager's Sub-office' and the surgical SHO on-call room you can find under 'Patient Pathway Discharge Facilitator Deputy Coordinator's Deputy Assistant Manager's Officer'.

Is this just my view? No. In October 2006 the Royal College of Physicians published a study *'Designing Safer Rotas for Junior Doctors in the 48-hour Week'* Its main conclusion was, 'Most junior doctors work night shifts, many of them are doing seven consecutive nights, each lasting 13 hours. That has been shown to be potentially the most dangerous type of rota that could be devised, in terms of risks to both patients and staff.' For futher information, please go to http://www.rcplondon. ac.uk/pubs/brochure.aspx?e=180.

Now that we know that the politicians have the evidence we shouldn't allow them to let hospitals arrange such dangerous rotas. The Labour government has brought about good changes to our working life styles but it needs to do more and do it faster – for the patients' sake. Change rotas now. It won't necessarily cost anything, it will just mean that medical staffing managers will have to think about things a little bit harder.

Oh, and one more thing on nights and sleeping: the seventh night of my week was very quiet – luckily. The nurses knew I had had a crap day and not slept that well and so I slept for an hour or two when it was very quiet. I slept in the side room where we often put patients when they are going to die, to give relatives some privacy. It was a little spooky – but needs must, especially when you are working a dangerous rota.

Changing emotions

It had been a very pleasant day at work. We were well staffed and everyone was in a good mood as someone had bought some Nescafé Gold in to replace the Happy Shopper coffee. How easily pleased we all are.

I picked up the next card: 28-year-old male. He hadn't been triaged yet so the only information I had was from the receptionist, who wrote 'not feeling right'. (I also knew his religion – for some reason they always find out the patient's religion. Maybe it is just in case we need some extra special help and it helps us to know who to call?)

I started chatting to him. He was a delightful man. He was there with his pregnant wife of seven months who had forced him to come. He started to tell me his symptoms. They were all a bit non-specific. He had felt tired and a bit sick for the last few days. I was about to advise him that he should have seen his GP instead when he added that he had tried to play the piano and it just didn't seem right. His hands didn't seem to touch the keys properly (he was a good jazz pianist apparently).

This concerned me. This shouldn't happen to 28-year-olds. I examined him and he had a neurological sign that concerned me – he couldn't tap his hands together properly. It worried me, first because it implied that he might actually have a brain tumour, and second because I had to write down such a long word in the notes that I would invariably spell wrongly – dysdiadokinesis. (Many doctors love medical jargon and long words because they think they are clever when they say them. I don't, partly because patients don't know what you are talking about, but mainly because I am shit at spelling.)

I left him for a moment to plead with the radiologists for a scan. After being told that I was probably wasting their time/ making up symptoms/exposing my patients to unnecessary radiation, they eventually agreed to the scan after I promised to sacrifice my first born child in their honour.

I explained to the patient that although the signs were probably caused by 'something minor' we had to rule out 'something more serious' going on inside his brain. He seemed satisfied by my explanations and went for his scan.

While he was in the scanner, all my colleagues were taking the piss out of me for organising another 'unnecessary' test and just looking for something dramatic to excite my day. I explained to them all why I believed he might have a brain tumour and went into detail about the anatomy of the damaged bit of brain. They explained to me that I needed to get out more and realise that most people's symptoms are caused by stress.

Just as I was saying 'I bet you he has got a tumour' and my colleagues were saying 'I bet you he hasn't', the radiologists called. 'You'd better come down and have a look at the scans.'

'Oh f**k', I thought, as I looked at the scan. But I am a professional and so collected my thoughts before contributing to the academic discussion about the scan results. 'Oh f**k', I said.

He had an obvious tumour. Not only that, but he had swelling of the brain and he would need immediate transfer to a specialist centre. This was the worst possible scenario that I could have imagined, but, strangely, from a purely academic point of view, I was pleased.

I was pleased that I had been proved right. Pleased that I had worked out his diagnosis from a weird set of signs and symptoms. But *de facto* I was therefore pleased that this man had a brain tumour with a possible death sentence. This is surely not right. I went to speak to my colleagues/doubters. A 'told you so look' went across my face as I told them what the scan had shown. However, as the glow of academic satisfaction dimmed, the reality struck. He had a brain tumour and would need an urgent operation tonight. He was seriously sick and might not see his child grow up... and I had to go and tell him.

It didn't go well. I told them what the scan had shown. He was stoical. His partner was hysterical. It was awful.

I left the conversation feeling sick. It had been a day of weird emotions: pleasure from an academic viewpoint and heartbreak from a personal one. It can be a very interesting job this one... but also very upsetting.

♺ Career stresses

There is a lot of uncertainty about working in A&E at the moment. In the past, to become a registrar, you had the stress of passing exams and having to move around the country for different jobs, but at least you knew that once you had finished your training, you could settle down as a consultant and help run an A&E department.

However, for the registrars of today's A&E, it is very different. More exams and constant revalidation, are things all specialist doctors should expect, but it is the uncertainty of what our role will actually be that is worrying.

Emergency nurse practitioners see a lot of the minor cases that doctors used to see. This was supposed to give us time to see the sickest patients. However, the government's 4-hour target is taking away our role in their ongoing emergency care (which is often beyond 4 hours) and it is being taken over by a new creed of doctors – acute medics.

Then there is the question of whether there will be jobs in the future for us once we have finished our training and are consultants. Hospitals are cash-strapped at the moment and there seems to be a reluctance to take on new consultants. Even the government has said that it anticipates that there will be too many consultants in a few years' time. Also, how many A&E consultants will we need in the future, if the government has closed all the smaller units?

So, if you see your A&E doctor looking stressed, it may be because of career worries on top of the other expected ones.

Bloody Jobsworth

Your job is hard enough and then you get twats making your job harder. They read protocols and policies, and then think they have power. I have had quite a few examples during my time as an A&E doctor. Here are a couple – the first one happened a couple of years ago.

It was a quiet night and I was the only doctor in a small A&E where everyone knew everyone else. At about 3 a.m. the knob of a security officer came over on his rounds. He was the type of security officer who instilled no confidence in either his fighting abilities or his conflict resolution skills. He was fat, greying and very sweaty and all he looked good for was making the tea for the post-fight analysis.

'Evening, Edwards,' he said in his quite irritating Birmingham accent. He walked off to check a door or something and then came back. 'Have you got your ID badge on you?'

'No.'

'Well, have you seen the new trust memo section 4, paragraph 6.2 section 3, line 7 on improving patient safety. It says if you have not got your ID badge, then you can't see patients and so I can ask you to leave.'

'Oh well… bureaucracy etc.' I responded.

'No, seriously, I could ask you to leave and I'll escort you off the premises if I want to,' he said.

'Look, just let me get on with my job and stop being pedantic,' I responded.

He retorted, 'I am just doing my job. I am not padantic.'

'Pedantic. Not padantic,' I responded, in what I thought

was a witty way, but he didn't get. 'I would be delighted if you escorted me off the premises. But who is going to see the patients?'

'Not my problem… section 4, paragraph 6.2, etc., etc.' He went on and on.

Now, I wouldn't have minded this conversation if he was joking, but he wasn't. He was deadly serious. I fought back in this game of verbal judo.

'Actually, please escort me off the premises, and you can explain why all the patients had to wait until the morning to see a doctor.'

He backed down, but then a week later I got a letter advising me about my section 4, paragraph 6 from the personnel manager and copied to my bosses. What a waste of NHS money and time.

But this wasn't as bad as the Jobsworth a colleague of mine got told off by. You may not have noticed, but recently the NHS has gone 'smoke free'. A great idea – no smoking in the building or grounds but a blanket ban lacks common sense. It is a fact of life that in A&E stressful things happen, and some people smoke for a bit of urgent stress relief.

A colleague of mine had been telling a dad about his 20-year-old son who had had a serious motorbike accident and had to go to ICU. The dad asked him if they could talk outside as he needed a cigarette. They went outside and carried on the discussion and my colleague explained in detail what was going to happen when his son was on ICU.

As they were talking, a health and safety manager, or something like that, walked past. 'You are not allowed to smoke in the trust grounds,' he said, while pointing to a ridiculously expensive, large banner draped across the outside wall of the hospital. My friend said he was trying to tell his patient's dad about his son's critical illness and asked him to leave them alone.

'Well, you can tell him without him smoking. We are a smoke-free site,' he said in a completely dispassionate way.

Ten minutes later the safety officer came back to tell off my colleague for encouraging members of the public to break health and safety regulations and advise him that if he did it again, it was a disciplinary offence. What a cock. People need to think about the problems people face when they come to A&E and think outside their own small box.

While I would never encourage smoking, in very stressful situations nicotine withdrawal can make the stress a hundred times worse. Don't make life harder for staff and patients/relatives. Rules need to be bent where appropriate.

Lack of staff

One way A&Es have adapted to the 4-hour rule is to bring in A&E-run observation units/clinical decision units (CDUs) for patients who are waiting for test results before they can go home or who only need a very short admission. They are not intended for people who are going to need admission regardless of the blood results. However, some hospitals don't have these wards, or perhaps only have a few beds, so patients are still needlessly admitted to the main hospital for a few hours.

Yesterday I found out how frustrating it must be to work in an A&E without these wards and with the government

4-hour targets. I was working on a day when our 'CDU' ward was closed because of staff shortages. I had a gentleman who had walked in from the street 10 minutes after taking 16 paracetamol tablets. The medical management for this is to measure the levels of the drug after 4 hours to see the level of paracetamol in the blood and then, depending on the level, to treat the patient with a drug to protect the liver. Absorption varies from person to person, so not everyone will need this treatment. It was unlikely that this man would need the treatment, but he would need to see a psychiatrist for his suicidal intention.

I wanted to admit him to our ward for the test so he wouldn't breach but I was unable to. He had to be admitted to the main hospital. He would then be seen again by the medical doctors, who would then take the blood and sort him out. Six hours after admission to A&E, they had his blood results and knew that, medically, there was nothing for them to do. However, he ended up staying the night as the medical team was unable to get a psychiatrist to come and see him as quickly as we generally can in A&E.

It was a waste of a bed, a waste of time for the medical doctors as they had to 'clerk him' (take a history and examine the patient) and a huge waste of money. The patient got the right treatment but was confused as to why he was being shipped around the hospital.

For me, it made me feel that my job was pointless. I am not on a training scheme to become a consultant in triaging patients. I am a specialist in emergency care. I didn't need to refer this patient to the medical doctors for their expert advice – it is my area of expertise. It really pissed me off.

Am I becoming sick?

Is it right that I am hoping patients have various ailments to make my job easier or more interesting? Surely the humanitarian side of me should want everyone I see to be pain- and illness-free? I don't and I am worried I should, but at least I know my thoughts aren't right…

Today I saw a little old lady who had a fall. She was living at home, and her carer had found her on the floor. She was confused and it was very hard to understand what had happened. On examination, I could tell that she had a painful hip. I sent her for X-ray and thought, 'I hope it is broken, because if it is, then she will be an easy referral to the orthopaedic doctors. If it is not, then I will have to do some thinking and sorting out.'

How wrong is that thought? I wanted to condemn the poor woman to an operation, weeks of hospital stay and a 30 per cent chance of dying in six months, just to make my job easier?

A couple of nights ago, I was getting quite tired and bored when I saw someone and sent them for a chest X-ray. I was concerned that they might have a pneumothorax (hole in the lungs). I was disappointed that they didn't. I wanted them to have that condition purely so I could get out of seeing another patient and put in a chest drain, which I enjoy doing. That surely isn't a right thought.

A few day before that, I was sure that I had seen a patient with a brain tumour. I was really proud of my clinical examination and history-taking skills. I sent her for an emergency CT scan and was disappointed to find out that she didn't have anything wrong with her brain at all. How wrong is that? (How can I be disappointed that someone hasn't got a cancer, just because it's lowered my confidence in my doctoring abilities?)

Do all doctors think that? Am I unusual? Am I an uncaring bastard? My fears were relieved at the pub when an anaesthetic colleague told me about her day at work. The ICU was full and there was a cardiac arrest on one of the wards. She ran down and during the resuscitation attempt, she kept on thinking, 'I hope she doesn't make it, otherwise I'll be up all night taking her to ICU. I want to go back to bed.' She then said how relieved she was that the resuscitation attempt had failed (although it had been conducted properly). She was relieved that a 60-year-old lady about to embark on her well-earned retirement had died, just so that she could get back to bed?

To someone who doesn't work in the NHS, these thoughts may seem very sick. But as long as you treat your patients to the best of your ability, regardless of any feelings, do not let patients know what you are thinking and realise that the thoughts are wrong, then what you are thinking deep down shouldn't really matter... I hope.

Why do we all lie?

One of the things that I have noticed working in A&E is the lies patients tell us. Perhaps 'lies' is too strong a word – I mean the things they say when they mean something else. Here are some examples I've had in the last few nights:

> *Patient says*: 'I didn't mean to bother you.'
> *Patient means*: 'I did mean to bother you.'

Patient says: 'I had a car accident two days ago and my neck hurts.'

Patient means: 'My unemployed mate who watches lots of daytime TV told me about "no-win, no-fee", no self-respect lawyersforyou.com and I think I am in for a fortune.'

Patient says: 'How do you spell your name?'

Patient means: 'You are getting a thank you letter.'

Patient says: 'How do you spell your surname?'

Patient means: 'You are getting a complaint letter.'

Patient says: 'I have got a personality disorder.'

Patient means: 'I used to be known as an attention seeker. Now I am medicalised by a hippy psychiatrist and you have got to be nice to me and treat my time-wasting seriously.'

Patient says: 'My drink has been spiked.'

Patient means: 'I got so drunk I need an excuse for my behaviour.'

Patient says: 'The GP told me to come/I tried for 2 hours to get a GP/The GP couldn't see me for two weeks.'

Patient means: 'I didn't bother to try and see my GP as I knew you would see me anyway.'

Patient says: 'I am an ex-smoker.'

Patient means: 'I gave up an hour ago.'

Patient says: 'You f**ker. You f**king f**ker. Why did you get me off my high you f**ker.'

Patient means: 'Thank you so very much for saving my life by giving me naloxone and letting me breathe on my own and stopping me being in a coma all my life after I overdosed on heroine.'

Patient says: 'I have been waiting over 2 hours.'

Patient means: 'I have been waiting 20 minutes but am in a rush.'

Patient says: 'I don't drink much.'

Patient means: 'I drink less than my doctor.'

Patient says: 'You won't break confidentiality with the police, will you?'

Patient means: 'I have been very naughty.'

However, there is not just patient to doctor lies; it's the other way round that I like best. Here are some things that I have heard some doctors say when I am sure that they might mean something else.

Dr says: 'This won't hurt.'

Dr means: 'This will hurt.'

Dr says: 'Don't worry, I have done this procedure loads of times.'

Dr means: 'Don't worry, I read about this procedure earlier today.'

Dr says: 'Emmm... I'll just be a minute.'
Dr means: 'I haven't got a clue. I'll have a look on the Internet for some medical inspiration.'

Dr says: 'So what accident or emergency do you have?'
Dr means: 'Why are you wasting my time?'

Dr says: 'I'll get a second opinion.'
Dr means: 'I still haven't got a clue.'

However, the ones I love the most are when patients actually tell the truth. Some recent examples:

'I have a carrot stuck up my arse. It helped me come and I like the feeling of it, but my wife is getting back from holiday tomorrow and Jason wants his carrot back.'

'My GP is shit and not giving me the answer I want, so I came to you instead.'

'I was lost so I called an ambulance as I live near the hospital. There is nothing wrong with me but I thought I'd come in for a check up as I am here already.'

The best honest comment I have ever heard was from one of our sisters who is slightly disillusioned by British culture...

Chaviest/ugliest girl ever: 'My drink has been spiked.'
Senior sister: 'I doubt it. People only spike your drink if they want to sleep with you.'

$\mathcal{Q}_\circ$ A typical day

So what is my average day like? Some people joke that it is same shit, different day – but the wonder of A&E is that the same shit comes in different colours and textures. I have chosen a random date to describe a typical day – my birthday.

I was doing a day shift, 8 – 6. Great, as it meant I that would see my wife and child in the evening, but shit because of rush-hour traffic on the way to work. The alarm went off at 6 a.m. and then turned onto Snooze a couple too many times. Quick shower and into the car – with a breakfast bar en route.

7.40 a.m. – arrive for the extraordinarily ridiculous hunt for the car park space. Find a spot and celebrate only to see that it is reserved for the hospital Chaplain (who rides a bike anyway).

7.55 a.m. – decide to park illegally by the back of A&E reserved for police and ambulance crews. Again, no spaces there as all my colleagues have done the same thing. Eventually, I park at the local DIY shop – I'll buy some screws on the way home from work, promise. Arrive 10 minutes late and stressed.

The first part of the registrar's morning job is to get a handover from the night doctor. After a quick assessment of the priorities in A&E, I delegate one of the junior doctors I have with me to see the two sicker patients. I then review the patients who were admitted to the A&E overnight ward – a combination of suicidal patients waiting to see the psychiatrist once they have sobered up, head injuries needing observations, little old ladies who have had a fall and need an occupational therapy assessment and the homeless alcoholic who was given a bed for the night.

Then it is off to see the minor patients – or patients that the triage nurse has deemed to be minor. You are expected to breeze through these patients and they usually require quick fixes such as a plaster cast or a few stitches. Unfortunately, some are far from minor and can take ages to sort out.

9.30 a.m. – the consultant emerges from his office, wondering why there are patients waiting: you either answer in a short-term view – that you have been caught up with a complicated patient – or you answer in a more socio-political way, i.e. there are increasing numbers of patients attending A&E without reciprocal resources, etc. Neither answer pleases the consultant and you are told to get on with it.

10.30 a.m. – have seen more minor cases and I am frustrated for a number of reasons:

1. When the emergency nurse practitioner is away on a course, why isn't there cover built into the rota and why am I just expected to cover the workload?

2. Why has the triage nurse let some of these patients through? A typical example is the toothache that has not been sent to the emergency dentist. So they wait for 2 hours for me to say, 'I am not a dentist – here is the number of the emergency dentist.'

3. Why have some patients come? Typical example – lump on leg for four years; have you not heard of a GP?

11.30 a.m. – just about to get a coffee and the 'red phone' goes off. This is the phone which is meant to tell us when sick patients are coming in, so we can get prepared. This time it was used for a patient who had had chest pain but now had resolved and who had a normal ECG. I got ready by drinking my coffee and taking the time to flirt with the nurse I will be working with. *The nurse flirts back and flicks her hair back and smiles at me.*

1.00 p.m. – lunch. Shit food. Not that cheap. Jamie Oliver, please come and look after us.

1.20 p.m. – *get asked out by the student nurse, aged 21, 34B, size 10.*

2–4.50 p.m. – see a few major and minor cases. Nothing that exciting happens, but what I do notice is the number of freaks that are coming in to see me. Too many freaks and not enough circuses I think. There are also lots of people who genuinely need my help and are appreciative. I like it when people say thank you.

***4.50 p.m.** – have to remind another nurse that I am married and she shouldn't try and snog me in the linen cupboard.*

5.00 p.m. – see an overdose. Fortunately, not that serious and I don't get that emotionally involved.

***5.25 p.m.** – turn down a come-on from one of the fit nurses.*

5.30 p.m. – department quite quiet, so I write a police assault form.

5.50 p.m. – persuade a heroin user that he shouldn't self-discharge after my colleague has reversed the effects of their smack, in order to help them breathe. Get told to f**k off.

6.00 p.m. – home time! Buy some screws in the DIY store and say I got lost in the timber section. Get the clamps removed from my wheels and go home as four ambulances rush by with major traumas that my colleague has to see.

So, while it can sometimes be a case of 'same shit, different day', it is a fact that no shit is like another and you never quite know what is going to happen next, which keeps my interest in my patients and my job. It is stressful, but time just flies past and at the end of the day I usually feel as if I've done something useful.

So all in all, a normal day with no major incidents, a few moans and a few pleasant patients.

P.S. Sadly, the bits in italics were all made up to boost my ego. The exciting, sexy things that you see on TV A&E dramas don't actually happen in reality. Sorry to destroy the illusion.

JFWDI

Contrary to what may come across in a lot of my rants at the pub/writings, I do not hanker after the good old days where the doctor knew best. They were bad old days. It led to arrogance in the medical profession and unaccountability. It is a very good thing that doctors have to justify their actions not only to themselves but also to the public and other professionals allied to health care – radiographers, biomedical scientists, etc.

Having to justify our actions to other health-care professionals, especially when we are organising tests, makes us think more about exactly what we are looking for and why. When we write request forms or phone up for an urgent test, we, quite rightly, always have to justify it.

Most other professionals know that sometimes the information you have can be sketchy, owing to the nature of

A&E work, and 99 per cent of staff are very helpful and get test results done as quickly as possible. Sometimes, however, that 1 per cent feels like 99 per cent. You feel that they have no inkling of the stresses of working in the A&E department when they are stuck in their fume-filled laboratories. You feel they sometimes follow protocol just to get out of work – and it can drive you mad. Here is a recent example of this.

I had a 43-year-old man come in to A&E. He looked dreadful, he had vomited blood and his heart rate was up but blood pressure hadn't fallen yet. My gut instinct was he needed blood – and quick. I fast bleeped the haematology technician, who slow responded. Five minutes later we got into a discussion on why I wanted blood when I hadn't got a result of his haemoglobin. (A pointless argument as, regardless of the result, he was going to need blood, or at the very least some standing by ready to be given just in case.)

Apparently the scientist in his lab knew exactly what was going to happen – even though he hadn't seen the patient. An unsuccessful discussion ensued and I was only successful in my argument when I asked for his name so I could write it in the notes and move the clinical responsibility to him. My blood then arrived quicker than you can say a short sentence quite quickly.

Why did I have to have a fight? I didn't ask for the blood just to piss him off, my patient needed it. I didn't want a stressful battle but I had to have one. Yes, he can question why I need the blood but in an emergency repeating an argument 10 times is not helpful to the patient or to me.

A few days previously to that, I had a patient who had been in a fight (a case of nasty walls again!). I wanted both the hand he had used to punch with and the elbow he fell onto X-rayed. Both were tender on palpation. An hour later, the hand X-ray came back – broken – but there was no elbow X-ray. I enquired as to why. Apparently, the radiographer didn't think it was broken and so didn't bother to X-ray it. However, I did think it *might* be broken and didn't want to miss a fracture. I take clinical responsibility for the patient and not the radiographer.

Again, I had to have a 10-minute argument about why I wanted to X-ray this man's arm. I didn't have the time for this. I tried to explain that the point of my being at work wasn't to upset diagnostic staff by getting them to do unnecessary tests, but to look after patients wanting (and occasionally needing) our help. Again, only by resorting to the 'What's your name so I can put it down in the notes, etc.' tactic, did I get my X-ray… which turned out to be entirely normal. I then got an episode of 'I told you so,' but at the end of the day it is my responsibility, so don't moan at me for being cautious and not wanting to end up in court for missing a fracture.

When the next pub opportunity arrived, I ranted about these episodes in a more and more manic way as the beer flowed (OK, I'll be honest, as the alcopops trickled). A friend of mine – also a doctor but much older and with years of experience – told me how he and his colleagues used to deal with these problems. They just wrote on the form JFWDI – it stood for 'Just f**king well do it.' This was before people questioned doctors. Few knew what JFWDI meant and so nobody would dare question the doctor. It is an amusing thing to write, but totally inappropriate. As I said earlier, I am so glad that times have changed – 99 per cent of the time.

At this point I want to say how totally reliant A&E doctors are on the other staff working in the labs/X-ray departments. They are usually highly skilled and, on the whole, highly efficient, helpful, frequently friendly and generally a pleasure to work with. It is just a small minority that drive me mad.

What these people lack is the respect and recognition for what they do – especially lab technicians and scientists. They have fallen behind the doctors' and nurses' pay scales and work hours that are often much worse than ours. However, unlike nurses – who are all apparently angels with a seat in heaven waiting for them – they don't get recognition and respect from the public, or politicians. An example I read in the paper was that a pop star wanted to say thank you for the care his mother had received in hospital. He was going to put on a free concert for NHS nurses. Great, but he didn't mention all the other NHS staff vital to making the place tick – lab scientists, physios, OTs, radiographers, secretaries, etc. And before you ask, doctors don't really need free tickets for pop concerts. Whatever anyone says, we are quite well paid and can buy our own tickets. I know very few really poor doctors. Lots of pissed off and stressed ones, but not many poor ones.

Male menstrual syndrome

I got really fed up at work this week. I tried to rationalise why and realise that my wife is probably right and I have got 'Male Menstrual Tension' – a little known condition but with symptoms far worse than PMT. It is often exacerbated by a lack of sleep, beer, sex and football – but nearly always induced by stress. It was the stresses and annoyances at work which set it off. These include:

1. The 4-hour rule – don't get me started.
2. The frequently rude patients that I have to treat.
3. The chav night club where the chavs go to for their chavy fights and then come to see me. N.B. When I go to the club, I tell people it is retro chic and not chavy.
4. Toffs with excessive expectations – there is only one little me.
5. People trying to kill themselves.
6. People trying to kill themselves but not very effectively – five vitamin pills will not do it but it will get you a bed for the night while we wait until the psychiatrist can see you in the morning.
7. Medical doctors. They moan a lot, can be arrogant and condescending, copy our clerking, complain that unnecessary tests have not been done and then say, 'Well I wouldn't have referred it.' Well then, you can send them home, professor. *Please note usually I don't think this of medical doctors and they are usually good colleagues – I am just having a bad week.*
8. Cardiologists who arrogantly say – 'So I suppose you want an unnecessary echo to make yourself feel better.'
9. Ophthalmologists who answer 'chloramphenicol' to every question.
10. Respiratory doctors who always ask if you have excluded TB. No! The test takes weeks. I only have 4 hours!

11. Out-of-hours GPs – don't get me started.

12. NHS Direct having no choice but to advise people to go to A&E to cover their own backs.

13. People coming in saying, 'I just wanted to get a second opinion.'

14. Drunk teenagers – when I was young I went home to sober up, not to A&E.

As I said, I am having a bad week. Normally I love my job but at the moment I am fed up. Sorry to be moody.

Delivering oranges

The next patient's card I picked up was an elderly lady, in her mid-70s with 'abdominal pain'. I quite enjoy seeing elderly patients. They are usually really grateful and undemanding, and you can always try and charm them. My favourite tactic is pretending that they must have given the wrong details to the nurse as their date of birth must be at least 10 years out. It always gets a smile and then the patient gets more relaxed. This didn't quite work with this patient. She gave a faint 'Don't be a patronising twat' smile and asked me if we could go into a private cubicle. I walked with her into the gynaecological room which has a door and some privacy. She started the conversation.

'I have an orange in my vagina, and I can't get it out.'

'OK. That's fine; I'll need to examine you to see if I can get it out. I'll go and get a nurse so that she can chaperone me. Don't worry, it's quite a common problem.'

What the hell was I saying? No, it wasn't a common problem, and what the hell was she doing with an orange in her fanny… and what was she doing not looking in the slightest bit embarrassed? She would have had the same facial expression if she had said she had slipped and fallen and hurt her wrist. I wanted to know how it got there, but I just couldn't ask. I just stood there pretending I was unfazed and unembarrassed. I always have to remember my medical ethics of being non-judgmental. I found a nurse, who was free to chaperone me.

'Don't ask any questions. Just stay with me in the room. I need a chaperone and some psychological support.'

She looked at me strangely but came with me into the room. I examined her and there was this large orange. There was no way I could get it out. If it had been a Clementine, or even possibly a Satsuma, I could have 'delivered' it. I explained to her that I couldn't get it out, but that it needed to come out, otherwise she could get a nasty infection. I told her that I was going to refer her to the gynaecologists, who were going to have to retrieve it under a general anaesthetic. She just nodded and said 'Thank you, doctor'.

I have never before written in the notes 'Diagnosis: orange in vagina'. But then in A&E you get to see lots of strange things.

The problems of alcohol

I am writing this after a Thursday night shift. There was a common theme running through most of the patients I saw – alcohol. Now I am not self-righteous or pious – I love a good drink and I am grateful to that drug for helping me flirt vaguely successfully over the years. However, what most people don't seem to realise, both the general public and law-makers, is that alcohol is a drug, and an incredibly powerful drug at that. It is addictive and a depressant, and it can really bugger up your body if used excessively. The reason people like it is that its depressant effects depress the inhibitory areas of the frontal lobe. In other words, it makes you think that you have actually got a chance with that really fit blonde, but unfortunately also makes you think that you should beat up her boyfriend to win her affections.

It needs to be used with caution... and then it can be brilliant. Unfortunately, people forget about the caution bit and the consequences end up at A&E. The short-term consequences are the fights, accidents and deliberate self-harm, and the long-term consequences are liver failures, the dementias and the suicides.

My shift started at 10 p.m. The first person I saw was a man who had come in after being forced to by his wife. He was in his 40s and had combined a career in business with a social life in the pub. He was the nicest man you could ever wish to meet. He was like Homer Simpson – funny, caring, devoted to his wife and children, and yellow. It was obvious that he was in acute liver failure – caused by the drink. Blood tests revealed his kidneys were not working either and that his liver was so damaged that as well as making him yellow, his blood couldn't clot properly.

The medical treatment isn't that complicated – once you have a diagnosis and a cause, you try and stabilise him, stop him drinking and send him to the ICU where they do expensive and clever stuff. Once patients go to ICU, it really is touch and go whether they survive, but the prognosis is usually very bad, especially if their kidneys are not working. I don't actually know what happened to this patient – one of the worst things about A&E is you don't get to follow up your patients. However, from experience, I wouldn't give him much of a chance. What a waste of life: a man in his 40s who should be spending time with his kids won't be because he spent too much time drinking.

The next patient I saw was a typical Friday night injury (I think Thursday is becoming the new Friday). He came in with a punch to his face and an injured little finger (known as a Boxer's fracture). I am not sure exactly what happened, but he mumbled something like: he went to the pub, got pissed, knocked into someone and spilt their pint. A 'What you looking at?' type of conversation started up. His mother was insulted and he questioned the other person's parentage. The final straw was that his sister's celibacy wasn't accepted as gospel by the person he bumped into. He had to defend the family's traditions and honour. He punched the bloke, who then punched him back, and, being a lot less pissed, the other bloke won the fight and left. My patient got the silver prize of an ambulance ride to A&E.

I examined him, and X-rayed his hand. His finger was broken, but the facial bones were normal. Now I don't really know why, but he didn't like this fact. I think he must have wanted them broken so he could press charges or something, and so when I tried for the fifth time to explain that he hadn't fractured his face, he called into question my masturbatory practices and implied that I f**k in a quite incestuous way (*for* *the record I have quite an average masturbatory practice and have a very conventional sex life*).

I had seen this bloke in the past and remembered that he was usually pleasant but this time because of booze, he had got himself beaten up and then become obnoxious. The time was only 10.45 p.m., so he had also ruined a potentially good night out. That was the second example of cautionless use of alcohol.

After grabbing a coffee, I saw my next patient. Some university students had been on a drinking binge all day, gone to a party and one of the girls had become so pissed she couldn't talk.

'She has had her drink spiked, she must have,' her friends informed me.

'So what has she drunk then?' I asked.

'Five double JDs and coke, five VOs and seven bottles of WKD.'

After deciphering the letters into drinks and then into units, I soon realised that I would be pissed on half of what she had drunk.

'She can normally handle her drink and so she must have had it spiked. Can't you do a test to prove it?'

I explained that this amount of booze will make you completely unconscious and that it is not usual to test for 'spiked drinks'. Her drink was already spiked with JD (Jack Daniels), VO (vodka and orange) and whatever alcohol they put into bottles of 'Wicked' (WKD).

The girl's night was ruined – she was so paralytic she wasn't bothered about the puke in her hair and didn't seem to care that she had wet herself. Our nurses' time was taken up by cleaning her up and my time was taken up by putting up a drip and giving her some fluids to help wake her up. Until she was safe and we were confident that she wouldn't choke on her own vomit, we had to keep her on a precious bed on the A&E ward with constant supervision. Because she so overindulged, our taxes paid for her to be cared for and she got a shit night. When she left in the morning, we didn't even get a thank you.

It makes you think that if booze wasn't so relatively cheap (especially alcopops and especially at university bars/drinks promotions nights), then she might not have the money to spend on this much booze, especially with tuition fees and the cost of shoes, etc. Maybe the government should think about increasing the price of booze, especially alcopops, as a deterrent to this sort of behaviour. I'll leave that to them and continue my recollections of last night.

While I was writing my patient notes, the 'red phone' went off. Ambulance control informed us that there had been a serious incident. A cyclist had been hit by a car doing 50 m.p.h. The cyclist was seriously injured.

I called the trauma team and the cavalry arrived – albeit a slightly bleary-eyed cavalry, moaning that they had been woken up and saying, 'I bet it is a load of bollocks – I want to go back to bed.' I arranged the team and got ready to lead them. The patient arrived a minute or two later.

It wasn't a load of bollocks at all. The ambulance men had done a brilliant job in getting the patient here so quickly as well as starting vital fluid resuscitation. But he was in a bad way. His heart rate was high and blood pressure low and his abdomen was rigid. (Coincidentally, my heart rate was off the scale, BP sky high and rectal continence indeterminate). He needed an emergency operation – no time for a CT scan. He needed his abdomen opening and the source of bleeding found and stopped. While explaining all this to him, all I could do was notice the stench of alcohol from his breath. This man was as pissed as a fart. No wonder he hadn't needed much analgesia. He was rushed to theatre and a bleeding spleen was found that had to be removed. He will now need life-long antibiotics, a week or two in ICU and weeks of intensive rehabilitation…oh, and a new bike.

The drink–drive message is starting to get through to people, but we seem to forget that it is also dangerous to drink and cycle. The majority of pedestrians injured in the evening have also been drinking and this may have contributed to their injury. Please remember this when you are running across the road after six pints – the green cross code still applies even if the kebab shop is about to close.

During the time it takes to run a trauma call, a lot of senior doctors and nurses are tied up and the other patients in the department end up having to wait a long time. The next patient had been waiting over 5 hours to be seen (3 hours 59 minutes in management timing). He was 16 and had gone over to his mate's house as he had a 'free house'. (Not a pub, but his parents had gone out for the evening.) He came in with his friend's parents after they found him vomiting (in their sock drawer for some bizarre reason) and because he couldn't walk straight or speak in a coherent manner.

They had initially tried to go to the pub, but first couldn't get served and second couldn't afford a pint anywhere except at the local Wetherspoon's and his granddad was there so he didn't particularly want to go in. They decided to go to the local supermarket with the friend's 19-year-old brother. Now I can hardly complain that he tried his best to obtain alcohol underage. I used to try every trick in the book – even resorting to brewing our own alcoholic drink in the local woods (you don't need to be 18 to buy yeast). But when I drank underage, I couldn't afford as much as this young lad could with his paper-round money. At the supermarket they managed to buy two packs of 20 bottles of Stella for something ridiculous like £14.99 – reassuringly dirt cheap, unlike the adverts would have us believe. These supermarkets are deliberately using amazing offers, potentially as loss leaders, to encourage people into their shops. This is ridiculous and just encourages excessive alcohol consumption.

The drinks industry doesn't approve either, because it is encouraging a form of drinking much worse than in a pub – isolated and without social interaction… or high profit margins. In the process the price war is causing local pubs to close. Can the government not stop this practice? I want more sensible red tape to protect the public. Why can't these supermarkets go back to their original loss leaders and sell baked beans for a penny, instead of shed loads of booze for not much?

Anyway, the young lad was examined and left to sleep it off till he was safe to go home. His parents then came in and I started to feel a little sorry for him – he got such a bollocking it was unbelievable, but also quite amusing.

So far it was five out of five patients who had been to A&E because of booze. The next patient I saw was an overdose. Yippee! Not an alcohol-related patient… except I had jumped to the wrong conclusion. He had taken a bottle of vitamin pills after drinking a bottle of JD (a very popular drink, I am finding out). The pills won't cause him any harm, but he needed a psychiatrist because he really did want to die and he thought the tablets would kill him. However, because he was pissed, no psychiatrist would see him until he had sobered up. He was someone else who was parked on a valuable observation bed for the night.

Six out of six became eight out of eight. Accompanied by the local constabulary two fine young members of the public had been brought in with various cuts and bruises. They had been to a local pub and got into a fight; police were called and then they were brought to us to get them checked out and stitched. Just so that the police wouldn't have to hang around for hours, I saw them promptly – no major injuries – just bruises. It was a waste of my time and it meant other more needy patients were not seen so speedily.

The pub in question is notorious – a new one built where I used to pay in cheques. They have also got a late licence – allowed by the government which is trying to encourage a continental café-style drinking culture and not a 'drink up, roll your sleeves up and fight' culture. However, at this new pub, they still have lots of heavy drinking and no one goes for a 'quiet coffee'. Why not? Well, the pub chains care about profit and not social responsibility and so to maximise profits they built a 'vertical drinking bar' as opposed to a French-style café. What this means is that you cannot sit down to have your drink slowly, the music is loud so you can't chat and there are no tables to rest your drink. So all you can do is drink till you get paralytic. If the councils just thought a little harder and granted late licences only to pubs that actually encouraged a café-style drinking culture (i.e. by having seats) then it might help with our booze problem. It is not a genius idea, just common sense.

Nine out of nine was a twisted ankle while running for a taxi, pissed, number 10 was a head injury after falling over, pissed, and numbers 11 and 12 were another fight (over who was looking at whose bird), pissed and pissed.

Reading this, you may think that I have a Presbyterian view of the new drinking laws – I don't. The 24-hour laws have, in my opinion, and that of a recent government report, not increased or decreased alcohol-related problems coming to us but just spread the workload over from what was originally 11 p.m.–1 a.m. to 11 p.m.–5 a.m.

The new rules have also done a lot of good. Police and local councils can liaise with the A&E departments about local problem pubs and they have been warned to buck up their ideas or lose their licences. The A&E consultants can also advise police and councils on safety issues. After consultation with one A&E department in Wales, a decision was made to force one pub/club to only sell booze in plastic bottles/glasses. The incidence of serious injuries decreased massively.

After an interval of three non-alcohol related patients I got my 13th booze-related patient: a Latvian builder whom I can only assume had misread the bottle label after work and drunk vodka instead of water (these mistakes do happen). He came in to ask if I could give him something to stop him vomiting and feeling so dizzy as he had to go and fix someone's roof soon! At least it won't be me who sees him when he comes back – it's my last shift for a few days and I am off to the pub now for a fry-up and a pint (the best bit about the new licensing laws).

✇ Upset at work

One case really upset me today. An old lady came in struggling to breathe. She was about 85. We tried all we could but soon her breathing stopped, as did her heart. We started CPR. Occasionally it works, but it was obvious in this case it wasn't going to work either: 15 minutes later, I checked with the team if anybody minded if we stopped. Nobody did. I went to speak to her husband.

'Is she dead?' he asked without emotion.

I nodded. 'Oh… what do I do now? I haven't been on my own for 64 years. May I see her?'

I tried to explain what had happened but he just wanted to see his wife.

He looked at her. 'I love you', he said, with tears rolling down his face he added. 'See you in Heaven,' and then he left.

It really upset me. However long you have done this job you do get upset. Also, you know that he will be back soon, as invariably widowed men die shortly after their spouses. I tried to get a cup of tea when the red phone went off and another patient came in – a chance for reflection was stopped by a multiple trauma.

My last thoughts

Today was my last day at work before a two-week holiday and the break from writing that would ensue. The main thing writing this book has done for me is actually to get me to think about what I do as opposed to just go through the motions.

As I drove home to the sounds of REM (who always put me in contemplative mood), I started to think about my job and day. Yes, I had had a good day. I had seen lots of varied and interesting cases (medical term for patients/people), ranging from a heart attack to a broken finger. I had seen a patient whose condition had really made me upset, but also made me thankful for what I have got. I had an email from a medical student thanking me for a teaching session I gave a couple of weeks ago, and positive feedback from my boss about a patient I had treated. I had flirted with the nurses, and patients over 80, and had had a good bit of banter with my colleagues.

So, all in all, it wasn't so bad a day. To top it off, we hadn't been worried about 4-hour waiting targets as we seemed to be well-staffed today. So, on a good day, I think there is no other job in the world that I would prefer.

On a bad day, well, that is different. The stresses of dealing with such heart-breaking cases can be hard to cope with. The nervousness about making a mistake and the worry that your treatment will do no good, are hard to live with. There is the paranoia of getting a complaint from a patient. Then there is the anxiety of a getting a bad reputation from your bosses for not managing the department efficiently or being thought of as shit by your specialist colleagues for not sorting out patients in the manner they deem appropriate. Combine all that with the worry of exams, revalidation and working your way up the career ladder when you now have no idea of what is waiting for you at the top, then it leads to a difficult job. However, I think the good bits outweigh the bad bits.

So, I think to myself, do I want to carry on? Well, yes I do. Hopefully, in a few years I'll be a consultant and, although that means more responsibility and extra challenges, it also means that I will have a voice and perhaps some power in trying to direct changes in an appropriate way as opposed to just being swept along with them.

Would I recommend being an A&E doctor to school kids, medical students and my own child? Yes... but only if they are mentally strong and can cope with the stress and upset involved in the job, only if they don't take criticism to heart, only if they have 'bouncebackability' (thank you for that word, Iain Dowie) and only if they can rationalize what is important in life and not get so stressed by problems of complaints, difficulties with management, and the uncertainty of their chosen career. If you are like me and possess none of these qualities, would I still recommend A&E as a career? Yes, as long as you have the love, support and compassion of a partner to help you through it all and support you when it gets rough. Luckily, I have the best possible one: Mrs Edwards, everything I do, you make do-able and worthwhile. Thank you.

♀ Apologies, acknowledgments, thank yous ℒ and hopes

It is unusual to start this type of ending with an apologies section. However, I think that it is probably wise. Very rarely have I mentioned the many colleagues (including many managers) who work very hard to help A&E departments function well and help provide good quality of care for patients. This is not because they are rare – far from it – they are the rule, it is just the exceptions that really drive me mad and make me write to vent anger. If a biased view has come across, then I apologise.

I have many thank yous to say. First, to the publishers for agreeing to sign a contract without seeing much of my work and just based on me ranting while having a tired cup of coffee after a set of nights. Second, to my agent for leading me through a process that I know so little about. I would also like to thank my friends for being supportive and listening to my rants down the pub.

I would like to thank all the staff I work with and the thousands of others who keep the NHS going. My particular thanks go to my recent immediate bosses for helping train me and showing how to keep your head when everyone else is moaning and ranting.

I would like to thank my family: my parents for their moral compass, my brother for his advice and my in-laws for encouraging me to write this book and giving me the idea in the first place. Most importantly, I would like to thank my wife. You have given me so much, including our precious child. This book has only been possible because of your support. Thank you. I love you so much. You have an unlimited shoe and handbag budget this year, I promise.

So that just takes us on to hopes and conclusions. I hope that you have enjoyed the book, and that it has opened your eyes to the reality of the subject material. I have shown you why I love my job and why it also drives me crazy. Generally, I think that things have got better in the NHS and emergency medicine in the last 10 years. The money pumped in has seen improvements. I think that the government's intentions have been right; it's just their actions that have been at fault. The problems have been the unintended consequence of poorly thought-out policies.

The NHS is an institution that I care about deeply. Policies have been brought in that tamper with its principles and ethos. I fear that the structural changes that have been brought in may lead to a patchwork privatisation and a consequential degradation in service provision. I hope a post-Blair era proves me wrong. If you too are worried, then try and do something to help save the NHS. We live in a democracy and our voices should count. Go on marches in support of the NHS, sign petitions, write to your MP or get involved with pressure groups such as the NHS Support Federation (www.nhscampaign.org). If you have any comments or wish to contact me please do so via The Friday Project or at drnickedwards@gmail.com.

Thank you.

Dr Nick Edwards, July 2007

Epilogue

Four years on and so much has changed. For me, personally, I have nearly completed my registrar training, including spending 18 months working as an intensive care doctor, to improve my skills with the sickest of patients in the resuscitation room. I have recently passed my fellowship exams and am now ready to apply for a consultant job. Sixteen years after starting medical school it will be great to stop being a junior doctor.

It hasn't been easy for my wife. We now have two kids under 4 and it has been hard for her with me having long commutes to work, studying for exams and having to change jobs every 6 to12 months. (She was also qualifying and working as a GP.) However, with the hope that in 6 months' time I will be a consultant with a fixed job and settled working pattern, things should be easier.

Things in A&E have changed for the better in the last 4 years. There have been more resources given to the NHS and emergency departments in particular. Through a dynamic and effective College of Emergency Medicine, the importance of A&E as a speciality is rapidly being accepted by hospital managers and politicians. There are more consultants than there were 4 years ago and more senior supervision of junior doctors – especially at the weekends and in the evening. Care has also improved. There is better treatment for strokes, heart attacks and trauma victims, more intensive care beds and a realisation that in conditions like septic shock it is the quality of the treatment we give in the first few hours that really affects patients' outcomes.

But over the last few years despite all the initiatives to reduce demands on A&E, more and more patients attend, expecting higher and higher levels of service. The pressures for the doctors and nurses on the shop floor have continued to rise. If I hadn't adapted my outlook, then there was no way I could have continued with the stress that this creates. I used to get so wound up by what I perceived as unnecessary micro-management, personal slights by other doctors or patients being rude and ungrateful. I used to come home angry after nearly every shift, but now I think my skin has thickened and I have realised what is truly important at work: how we care for our patients.

I have chosen a few stories to highlight what working in A&E during these last few years has been like. The important bits: working with colleagues, the satisfaction you can have from treating patients and the despair when our care doesn't work. It is not just a barrage of moans. Most importantly I have tried to show the amusement that work can bring and why there is no other job that I could do.

The problem with French

'Je m'appelle Nick. Je suis votre docteur. Vous êtes à l'hôpital.' The basic French that my mum had fastidiously taught me was at last becoming advantageous. The patient I was currently talking to was a Frenchman in his 20s. He currently had a tube in his windpipe which was helping him to breathe following a drug overdose of GHB.

GHB doesn't often hit the headlines but can very dangerous; a small bit makes you horny, a bit more euphoric, and just a tiny bit more completely unconscious and unable to breath unaided. This was what happened to this particular gentleman at a local nightclub a couple of hours previously.

But now the drug was starting to wear off. He was starting to wake up and the breathing tube needed removing. For it to be done safely, it needs to be done with full cooperation of the patient and without them being stressed. I had found a French ID card in his wallet and thought speaking in his native tongue would help calm him down, especially as he couldn't talk to us with the tube in. But it just seemed to make him more stressed.

When we had taken out the tube he started to scream in French: 'What the hell am I doing in France? I went away for a weekend party in England and now I am here. What the hell has happened?'

My French wasn't good enough to translate that I was just trying to help, and so I spoke in English from then on. He was much happier after that.

Not good enough for some people

With the increasing use of the internet and such wide-ranging reporting of medical issues, I sometimes feel in competition with the patients as to who has the most medical knowledge. This was exemplified by two slightly tipsy patients who had got into a fight. One of them had sustained a nasty forearm laceration which needed exploring in theatre under anaesthetic to check in case there were tendon injuries. His friend entered into the room – uninvited, I may add – voice first. I took an instant dislike to them – it saved time.

'Just stitch his wound and we'll be off,' the friend slurred. I looked at the patient and was trying to explain what I needed to do when his friend butted in and proffered more advice. 'He'll need some ice an' all.'

'Oi love,' he bellowed to the nurse. 'Fetch us some ice will, ya?'

Turning to me he gave some more scientific explanation to his advice. 'Slows down blood clotting, you see. He don't need an op, just stitches or a bit of glue.' At this point he fell off his stool. He sat there and continued to slur, and mumble general advice at me.

The only thing worse than a patient talking crap, is a patient's friend speaking utter crap. I tried to explain why just stitching up the wound would be a very bad idea. Neither listened. They both continued to talk drunken gibberish and irritate me.

The next question really blew me away.

'Anyway who are you to tell me what I need to do with my arm?'

I took a big breath about to list my many years' study, various letters after my name and degrees I have, when he rendered it all moot by declaring: 'My mate has a first aid at work certificate and he says stitch it and so stitch it.'

Again I tried convince him this was not the best course of action when he proudly announced he was off home to stitch it himself so he could get back to the pub. With that he self-discharged, although he did accept a bandage to stop it bleeding. A village was about to get their idiot back but only for a few hours.

Five hours later and a bit more sober, and after a good telling off from his mum, he came back and apologised. Exploring the wound showed a severed tendon which needed a plastic surgeon to repair the next day.

Two important things to remember here – just because a patient wants something, doesn't mean that we should and must do it. They are patients and not customers. Customers may always be right, but patients certainly aren't. But far more importantly I realised that if you find these types of interactions stressful, then you can't do A&E for a career. Luckily I enjoyed every minute of my time with this man.

Dealing with death

Some things I find very hard to cope with at work. It had been a fairly boring and standard Saturday afternoon shift. Then the 'red phone' went off and the horror call came in.

'Twenty-two-year old male. Cardiac arrest. CPR in progress. No return of rhythm.'

A call was put out and the team arrived. A friend of mine, Mike, came down from anaesthetics to help in case there was a problem with the patient's airway. He started to make jokes. This is quite normal when waiting for a patient – it helps relieve some tension. But this occasion was different. I told the story and he shut up.

The patient was a semi-professional Afro-Caribbean rugby player. He had suddenly collapsed in a cardiac arrest mid game, in front of a couple of thousand spectators. The team physio had rushed on and immediately started heart massage. When the paramedics arrived they told us that they could hear a pin drop in the stadium. They had been working on him for 40 minutes but nothing they had tried had managed to restart the heart.

The waiting arrest team descended on him as he came through the doors to resus. Drug after drug was given to try to kick start the heart back to life. Everything we could think of: more adrenaline, some atropine and calcium gluconate to help correct possible electrolyte imbalances. I did a scan of his heart, but there was no obvious cause for the arrest. It just wasn't beating. Emergency blood tests called a 'blood gas' showed the situation was a dire as it looked – the results were incompatible with life.

Just then his girlfriend arrived. One of the nurses led her into the corner of resus as she wanted to watch what was happening. She calmly stood back, saying nothing, but with tears rolling from her eyes. This man, her boyfriend and father to her child, was clearly dead but we continued on as we wanted to show her that all was being done to try to save him. It was all an act as everything proved futile. Eventually I think she realised this too.

I told her we were going to stop. She just nodded. Everyone was in agreement and resus went from a hive of noise and frantic activity to complete silence as we stopped. This poor man in the prime of his life was dead.

I had seen death many times, and been affected by it before, but this time it was surreal. It was like I was watching down on myself being in charge, detached but still focused. I knew there wasn't anything more that the team could have done.

I did what was necessary. Called the coroner, certified the body and had another chat with his girlfriend. I soon learned that his parents hadn't been told and that a colleague was trying desperately to contact them. In the waiting room was an anxious rugby team desperate to find out what had happened to their friend and teammate. I asked to speak to the manager alone, but he wanted me to tell all of them together what had happened. Oh boy, I thought, and took a deep breath.

I cleared out our coffee room of staff and rubbish and lead them in. A few burst into tears. One asked if he could see the body. Then another and then another. Then they all decided they wanted to see him and so they were shown into resus in pairs.

Meanwhile my colleague had got through to his parents and informed them; they were due to arrive in about half an hour. I wrote up my notes and started to see another patient as the department had become so busy. As much as I wanted to stop and collect my thoughts, life went on and there were patients to see. A nurse came to get me when the parents arrived.

Walking back into resus I was astounded by the sight that greeted me. His mum was screaming at his lifeless body, wailing and slapping his face and jumping up and down. It was almost a chant and unlike any form of expression of grief I had ever seen up until now. I am used to a western type of mourning, which is often rather quiet and reserved as relatives sit in stunned silence.

'Wake up. Wake up. Wake up.' She seemed to scream this for ages and ages. With the pitch getting louder and louder and her voice more and more frantic I had to interrupt and try to calm her down. I introduced myself. I explained what had happened and that there was nothing more we could have done.

She looked at me with anger and pushed my chest before starting to scream again, but this time it was: 'You killed my son. You killed my son. You killed my son.' The screaming at me, the screaming at her son and the physicality of her mourning seemed to go on for ever. I felt helpless at even beginning to aid to her cope with her grief. As more of the patient's family arrived, similar chanting and wailing echoed though the department. As uncomfortable as I felt and as unused to this form of grief as I was, my discomfort was nothing compared to what his family went through. I led them back to the staff coffee-room and let them get it out of their systems. Everyone and every culture have a different way to deal with grief.

A guide to A&E sisters and charge nurses

If you are ever in the 'majors' part of A&E, I am sure you will agree that it looks like organised chaos. But I assure you, there is method in the madness. This attempt at order is usually down to the senior nurses who run the department. They take the handover from the ambulance crew, they coordinate their staff, liaise with the senior doctor about what is happening to various patients, make sure patients are being seen on time and keep managers abreast of what is happening and often have to fend off irate relatives who feel they are being left too long to wait. It is a thankless task.

I have now worked in many hospitals and with many senior A&E nurses and have come to realise that there are a few stereotypical types of A&E nurse with various management styles. They usually conform to these stereotypes except for one mad sister who managed to encompass all styles in a single shift. Sometimes in a single sentence.

> **The Fat Controller** – like in Thomas the Tank Engine, the Fat Controller reigns supreme. They are fat because they have a chair with wheels. They rule with an iron fist and control everything including the chocolates and biscuits. They bark orders and manage well, but don't seem to be able to get off the chair. Often they get on very well with the registrar doctor – we also like to sit in a chair and 'direct'. But they are tough and when the going gets tough, they sit and tell you their tales from how much worse it was when they worked in another inner city A&E.

> **The doctor nurse** – known as a noctor –'Doctor, will you go and see the bloke in cubicle 3. He has got heart failure. I have given him GTN, morphine and frusemide. You need to sign for them. I have bleeped the medics for you… Oh here you are, they are on the phone.' That is one way of dealing with a very junior

doctor, but I have heard the same conversation with consultants. Their management style can be loved by managers as it means patients are processed out of A&E very quickly, but sometimes patients present with symptoms out of the box where a set recipe is not the best treatment.

The coercive – somehow with their personality they make people do things for them. A busy ambulance team arrives. They have handed over the patient. The Coercive flicks her hair back. 'Oh you wouldn't mind just taking them to cubicle 3 and attaching them to the monitor. We are all one seamless team, you know. I hear you are wonderful at doing bloods – you couldn't just do a quick set on him could you? Tea, white and one sugar please – my cup is the blue one. Thanks darling.' It's those two words – thanks darling – which help them get away with it. 'Can you just work that bit harder, stay an extra couple of hours and not have any breaks... Thanks darling.'

The rude ones – they just bark orders. Never smile. Slag off everyone and everything. They often combine their personality with a desire to be seen as above board as possible and so spend hours writing copious notes and incident forms in case they get in trouble.

The manager's pet – desire to fulfil targets is greater than desire to care for patients. These are the type of lead nurses who can really wind you up. You are half way through looking after your patient when nature calls. You return to the patient, but they have already taken over and referred them to the medical team and moved them to the ward. They also put unreasonable demands on the junior doctors – 'They have been waiting nearly 4 hours and so you have only 10 minutes to see them, make a plan and either admit or discharge them. I don't want them hanging around in my department. And before you ask – no, no one can do your bloods for you.' They love to use the word 'escalate'. Doing a night shift with this type of lead nurse is often a harrowing experience.

The generally lovely – nice, kind and warm to everyone. Helpful to the doctors but not dictatorial. Oozes experience and compassion. Manages their team well. Makes sure the department and patients are safe. Thinks about the patients first. Comes in various forms – some are more laid back than others, some are a bit obsessive and others might get a bit stressed, but they all have the same essential qualities. Luckily, the vast majority of senior A&E nurses are like this. Just a shame that they are underpaid, overworked and underappreciated. To the scores of top quality A&E nurses, thank you for making my job that bit easier. Now can I have the last choccie biscuit please?? Darling?

Abnormal observations

It happens every other Tuesday and one weekend in seven. If I refer a patient to the medical team with bradycardia (low heart rate) or hypotension (low blood pressure), and if they are then seen by a particular medical junior doctor, then, within a couple of minutes, the patients' observations miraculously improve. Heart rate and blood pressure up and I look like a fool who can't do simple patient observations. A sub-analysis of the patients who respond this way show it is 96 per cent of male patients and about 3 per cent of female ones.

The explanation for this is wonderful but wrong. This particular house officer (now called a Foundation One doctor: FY1) is dressed more in keeping with being a foundation one stripper. She is pretty, very pretty – 5 foot 9, long blonde hair, beautifully made-up face, manicured nails and a size 8. That is fine, but it's what she is wearing that causes such dramatic improvements in some patients' observations. She dresses very professionally. Well... professionally for an escort perhaps. Usually black high heels, or perhaps knee high stiletto boots, a short skirt which finishes a few inches below her knickers and the tightest of T-shirts. To top the look off, there is a stethoscope swinging gently across her overexposed breasts.

Now, don't get me wrong. I love this look and it makes my day when she comes down to A&E. All the boys' eyes just follow her around for a couple of minutes and we all enter a slight trance as our daydreams run away with us. As lovely as she looks, it is completely distracting and very unprofessional for a doctor. As much as all the ladies would enjoy it if I were to see patients in a tight T shirt, with my six pack bulging, wearing only tight Armani underwear, showing my perfectly formed posterior and my more than ample manhood, it would not be right. It gives the wrong impression and completely undermines what she is trying to do as a doctor.

I and most of my colleagues wear scrubs, which in the days of hospital acquired infection are more hygienic, they easily identify who I am and what job I do and allow patients and colleagues concentrate on the job in hand. I know it would make my days less enjoyable but I really think it is time all doctors working in the wards or in A&E started wearing a uniform like the nurses do.

But going back to our heroine of the day – I might ask her to keep her preferred attire close by, just in case we have a very sick patient whose blood pressure doesn't respond to the usual dose of fluids and drugs and needs an urgent extra tonic.

Good form of pre-op anxiolytic

It was a Friday evening when I saw a young lad who had crashed his motorbike. He was a bit upset generally, rather unhappy that we had to cut his clothes off and apoplectic that he was in hospital. He kept announcing that he was 'Outa here.' Sadly he wasn't going anywhere. Not for a long while.

We did the usual emergency medical treatment indicated in these sorts of cases: strong painkillers which had the added effect of calming him down, and cleaning the wound properly before getting him X-rayed. His X-ray showed a nasty fracture of the tibia bone. As it was an open fracture (a break which is exposed to the outside world via the cut), he would need it operated on quite quickly or risk losing the entire leg due to infection.

He was quite nervous about the operation and a general anaesthetic. I told him it was much safer than riding a motorbike and he needed to try do everything that he could think of to relax. I left him pondering this and got on with the rest of the shift. I didn't think about him till later in the night when the orthopaedic registrar came and spoke to me.

'What did you tell that young lad?' he enquired curiously. He went on to tell me that when he went to see him, and opened the curtains, that he interrupted his girlfriend providing fellatio to him. The young lad's response was that the A&E doctor told him he needed to do anything to relax and this was the best he could think of. The orthopaedic registrar left and scrubbed out the pre-op sedation from the drug chart. It wasn't really needed now.

Broken leg

The ambulance phoned ahead to say that they had a 12-month-old baby girl coming in with a broken femur (top bone of the leg.). This is a rather unusual fracture in a child, especially in a 12 month old. It takes rather a lot of force to break the thigh bone, and it would be very unusual for this to happen in a child by accident. The minute the call came in everyone was concerned that this was caused by a deliberate action from an adult – child abuse

The mother came in – she looked like a child herself and didn't seem to realise the enormity of what was happening to her child or that we would be looking closely at her story.

In these sorts of cases, the parent's history when compared to the physical injuries is paramount and both need to be carefully recorded. No one wants to unnecessarily accuse a parent/carer of abuse but then we also don't want to miss anything and risk further harm occurring.

Since cases like Baby P and Victoria Climbié, all health care professionals have regular teaching on how to spot 'non-accidental injuries' and it is often at the forefront of our minds in cases like this.

I sat down with the mother and tried to go over how her daughter had become injured. According to her she had stood her up on the nappy changing table and the leg just snapped.

The likelihood of this being true was quite low. Her story also seemed to have several inconsistencies especially about who was present when the accident happened. One minute one of her friends had been there, then just her boyfriend, then the next minute no one else was there.

X-rays showed the baby had what is called a spiral fracture of the thigh. Instead of a clean snap across the bone, the fracture was twisted just as if the leg had been twisted. Careful examination of her body also revealed some bruises that were clearly made several days ago as well as some small scars that were possibly cigarette burns.

Throughout this whole exam the baby just wanted her mummy. I don't know what had actually happened to the baby. We still don't exactly and maybe never will. Maybe the mum's boyfriend had hurt the baby and lied to her and she had just retold the story. Maybe she had twisted the leg in a fit of anger as she couldn't cope. I don't know. What I did know is that I had grave concerns about the safety of this child and the family situation.

We admitted the baby and she went up to the paediatric ward where again the paediatricians examined her and listened to the mum's story. Duty social workers were contacted and they and the police needed to do the full investigations to find out what truly happened and if the child should be removed from its family or put on the 'at risk register' and carefully monitored.

Throughout this whole case I felt sick to the depths of my stomach. She was about the same age as my daughter and looked quite similar. How could someone have done this to a poor defenceless baby? Who could hurt a child? Why should this child be treated so badly when my one is just spoilt rotten? And worst still, why is not just an isolated case, but rather an increasingly frequent occurrence in my line of work?

Nice bum

It was a busy Thursday night and walking into the waiting room was like being a gladiator, choosing which animal you would fight with next. All the usual A&E suspects were there – drink, drugs and plenty of fighting. I couldn't cherry-pick whom I could see, and just picked up the next card.

On this particular night there was one female patient waiting to be seen. Every time I went into the waiting room, she would try to catch my attention in order to jump the line. Usually her tactic would be to embarrass me by shouting, 'Oi sexy. See me next, doc.' What she didn't know is that I am generally immune to embarrassment and I ignored this banter and got on with the job.

However, each time I went into the waiting room she got a bit louder and feistier and the waiting room got a bit more information as to why she was there.

'Mr. Smith please,' I would say.

'Oh darling, Yes, you sexy doc – my bum's bleeding!' she would tell everyone.

Ten minutes later, 'Mr Jones please,' I would call.

'Come on sweetheart. See me next. The dog bit it'

This went on a bit longer till I called another patient. 'Mr Andrews ple—''

'For f**k's sake... Just have a look at it and tell me if I need stitches.'

In the middle of the waiting room, she proceeded to whip up her skirt, bend over and give everyone a good look at her ample derrière that had a small scratch on one cheek. Not really a good reason to be moved up the queue. I carried on seeing Mr Andrews who limped into minors on his twisted ankle with a slightly glazed, happy expression.

'Do you know what, doc? I feel better already,' he said.

The power of the mind, or not

Some people are not fans of western medicine and we must respect their wishes. A few months ago I had one. She was an odd lady, kept on insisting on telling me she was a feminist who had gone to prison for her beliefs. (She looked like a lady who definitely should have been put behind bras, but not necessarily in jail.)

She had sustained quite a nasty fracture to her wrist and it needed pulling into a straight position. I told her I wished to put local anaesthetic into the fracture and give her some sedation and sort her out.

She insisted that she only wanted natural treatment. She had never taken a tablet, immunisation, an injection or anything which can harm the body, which was odd considering she smelt of tobacco, but hey ho.

I tried to explain the need for the repair of the injury. She said she understood and asked me to go ahead and proceed in 10 minutes when she was 'prepared'. I was warned again that she must not be given any drugs.

I continued to persuade her. I failed. She insisted that I manipulate the fracture when she had prepared the mind. After trying to convince her of just how painful this procedure would be with out appropriate painkillers, I reluctantly agreed. I had no option. She was well within her rights to refuse painkillers.

She asked if she could play some music – I had no objections. Whale noises started coming from the iPod. She then started to close her eyes and rhythmically chant. This was going to be amazing. I had heard of the fire walkers and others who put mind above matter but never seen it before. A case report in a journal beckoned. I could retell her story. I started to get quite excited about what I was about to witness.

She raised her left arm, the signal we had agreed when she had prepared her mind. I gripped her fracture, content in the knowledge of her mystical powers and that this was the first non-urgent fracture that I would manipulate without analgesia. And then as I went to move the break... She screamed like she had never screamed before and I had never heard before. The whole A&E department was silent except for the screams.

'Give me the drugs now. I want the drugs. I need drugs. I couldn't give a damn about polluting my body. Drugs, drugs, drugs.'

Just then my boss walked in. 'Give her what she wants, Nick', and off he walked content that he could mock me to our colleagues.

℞ Why wanking turns you blind

A 60-year-old man walked into A&E.

He complained of sudden onset headache during the process of masturbation. It was like a sledge hammer to his head, he said. He had been sick once and was a bit confused.

On examination he was generally well, but with some neck stiffness. There were no hairs on his palms.

An urgent CT scan showed a bleed on the brain – a specific type of bleed called a subarachnoid haemorrhage with extension into an intracranial haemorrhage (a type of 'stroke').

He developed left-sided weakness and a blindness on the left side. He was soon stabilised and referred to the neurosurgeons for them to try to stop any further bleeding.

What had happened was that this man had a ticking time bomb, a small aneurysm (outpouching) of a blood vessel, which was liable to bleed by anything which put up his blood pressure. It just so happened that the thing which put up his blood pressure was self-gratification.

So you can see for this case that a stroke lead to a stroke, and that wanking can really turn you blind. I doubt that is going to put many men off but it's always good to have all the facts!

Teaching at every opportunity

One of the things I love to do is teach. This is probably, though, because I like the sound of my own voice and I can pretend I am on stage doing stand-up. I had agreed to give a talk to 20 medical students at the hospital as part of their preparation for their final exams. A very big deal to medical students who at that stage of their careers are in a mass panic and gladly grab any offer of teaching with two hands. I liked doing it and wanted to help them as much as I could. Even though my wife was pregnant with my son and was due around that time, I was confident I could make the time and help them out.

Early that morning, however, my wife's waters broke and mild contractions started. 'This is it,' we thought, all excited to meet our new son. I called grandma to come and babysit our daughter, got her an endless supply of 'Peppa Pig' DVDs (for my daughter, not my mother) and drove my wife to the hospital. While my wife was booking in, I called the medical school secretary to apologise. There was no one else able to give the talk and so they put up a note cancelling it.

When we arrived she was only 3cm dilated and the contractions had all but stopped. So we were advised to go for a walk for several hours to get things moving again. Fun as this sounds it was actually quite dull and I was feeling peckish so I convinced my wife to go to the hospital canteen for a fry-up breakfast. Obviously my wife couldn't eat much as she was in labour and didn't fancy it, but I thought it important that I keep up my strength for possibly a long day. By the time I'd eaten and read the morning papers it was still only 9 a.m.

and it was clear that not much was happening with the baby. Another circuit around the local park and we were both fed up.

'Well, as not much is happening shall I see if any of those med students are around still and you could sit at the back and learn what to do for patients in respiratory emergencies?' I asked brightly, thinking this was a great solution. Strangely my wife seemed a bit upset by this idea but I put it down to the hormones.

Thirty minutes later the lecture was back on, with many of the students having hung around and more than happy teaching was back on. They did seem to think it was a bit odd that there was a heavily pregnant woman sat at the back, sweating and moaning repeatedly. But the lecture went well I thought. Back on the labour ward things had sped up again and only three hours later I was clutching a beautiful baby boy. It was then pointed out to me that this might have been a bit self-centred to take teaching in the middle of my wife's labour but everyone was happy in the end. Weren't they?

Why being a doctor outside work isn't always good

Sometimes it is best off not mentioning you are a doctor. A National Childbirth Trust (NCT) meeting is one of them. So that we could meet other new parents in the area, we attended six two-hour antenatal sessions in the run up to our first child's birth. These classes were designed to prepare us for the birth and answer any questions as well as introducing us to other parents-to-be in our local area. It was my wife's idea. I went with it.

The classes were torture. Each week I would come back with more and more bruises on my upper arm, from my wife's elbowing me to be quiet, and with blood in the mouth from all my tongue biting. NCT classes are very good and informative but we both felt they had a slight anti-medicine slant; all about natural home births are best and no medical interventions and just what horrible things doctors would do to you if things started to go wrong. While well meaning and true in some aspects it was not good to hear when you are a doctor and have repeatedly seen what 'hospital medicine' does to save the lives of mums and babies during childbirth. At the penultimate meeting, I couldn't control myself. They were talking about vitamin K after birth for the newborn baby. This is a vitamin that is given routinely to all babies in the first day or so after birth to prevent those who are deficient in vitamin K from suffering bleeding on their brains. It is a treatment which saves lives throughout the world, is cost effective and evidence based. However, our class leader was trying to inform us of the side effects but seemed to be using tactics that scared more of the class rather than reassure us all. We were told to think very carefully about having it as the dose given to babies was very high and was it more than they really needed. We were then asked why we thought that dose was given.

I couldn't help myself. 'That's the dose given because that's the dose that all the evidence and safety data have shown is safe for babies and is effective enough to saves lives. Yes, it means giving an injection to a newborn baby but personally I would prefer to have an unnatural "medicalised" birth with mum and baby who are alive and well at the end of it rather than a natural birth and a dead baby and possibly mum at the end of it!' There was silence throughout the class and the instructor hurriedly changed the topic. The bruise from my wife was enormous and was still there when my daughter was born a couple of weeks later. Despite a few differing attitudes to childbirth, we made some very good friends in that class whom we still see four years later. We all had healthy babies and no one (well, possibly my wife still) seemed to mind my outburst.

Cheeky patient

It was 10 a.m. in the morning and I called the cardiology on call doctor.

We had quite a sick patient in A&E with an irregular and fast heart rate – atrial fibrillation. He was running at a rate of 200 and, at the age of 69, it was putting some dangerous pressure on his heart and he was suffering severe pain.

He needed to be 'shocked' out of his abnormal rhythm. For that you need two doctors, one to put him to sleep – the job I was going to do – and a second doctor to time the defibrillator to deliver the electric current and shock his heart back into a normal rhythm.

I was setting up my drugs while the cardiologist was chatting to the patient trying to find out more of a history. However, he wasn't getting very far as he was being repeatedly called away by other wards paging him. At first he ignored it but then realised it might be important.

The ward nurse apologised as they knew he was busy and they had already contacted him about the same thing twice but things were heating up. A 65-year-old inpatient who had had an angiogram (investigation of his heart blood vessels) in the morning wanted to go home asap. He had started kicking up a fuss about the waste of time he was having. The nurses had explained that the doctor needed to come and discuss the results with the patient but that he was busy. The patient had insisted that the nurse phone my cardiology colleague again.

The conversation was short. Twenty seconds and a few muttered swear words later, he was back with our very sick patient.

'I am ready to go, Nick' he said. I slowly injected the anaesthetic, a white fluid called propofol – often referred as 'milk of amnesia' – and off the patient floated into a world of sleepiness.

We shocked his heart. No effect. Our heart rates went up. His, however, didn't change. The cardiologist's bleep went off. He ignored it.

We shocked him again and his heart paused. Two anxious seconds left it went back into another rhythm – but not normal. His bleep went off. He ignored it.

We shocked him for a third time. This time it worked. His heart rate went back to normal. The cardiologist's bleep went off again. It was an outside line and he went to answer it.

'Hello, there my name is Mr Smith. I am on the cardiac ward waiting to be discharged. Do you mind pootling down to see me. I am awfully busy tomorrow and want to get home in good time...'

He went on, 'I am calling from those new patient line phones – switchboard kindly put me through, I said you wouldn't mind...'

I only wish I could put a picture of my colleague's face in the book. It would paint a thousand words.

What patients have taught me

As doctors, we often forget that encounters with patients often end up teaching us quite a lot of lessons. Here are a few of mine.

Never using a euphemism for death

A colleague went to tell the relatives of a 70-year-old man, who had died from a car accident, well... that he had died. Except he didn't use the words dead or died. He said that he had gone to a better place. The family just nodded and so to give them some time to be alone and grieve, he quickly left the room. The family came out five minutes later asking for the directions for the local trauma centre, as that is what they thought of as a better place.

We should change the way that we teach juniors

I saw a patient who needed a chest drain for an accumulation of fluid in his lungs. I had performed this procedure many times before and wanted to teach a junior colleague what to do. I asked the patient, expecting a 'yes of course doctor, three bags full doctor' style of answer, but when I told him that it would be the junior doctor's first drain he said: 'Would you go on an aeroplane where the pilot had not practised on a flight simulator first?'

Initially I was annoyed, this doctor had to learn, but then I realised that the patient had a great point and that simulation is something we should do as students before being let loose on patients. However, nothing makes up for the real thing and we are all eternally grateful for those patients that do let us hone our skills on them.

Being honest with patients

I used to get flustered seeing patients with whom I didn't know what was wrong. But after one encounter I learned to realise that being totally honest is the best way. I didn't know what was wrong with this 45-year-old lady and tried to tell her, but was failing badly.

'Be honest, you haven't got a clue what is wrong with me,' she said. I meekly nodded. 'Which is bad because I still don't know what is going on with me, but must be good as you know all about life-threatening conditions and I assume this is not one of them?' 'Yes,' I replied. I now use a variation on what she said and I think patients appreciate the honesty.

Being personal

I was having a discussion with a dad about what to do about his child who had fallen off a horse, sustained a head injury and who had vomited twice. I explained that we could scan his head and see if there was any injury but this would mean exposing him to potentially unnecessary radiation, or we could watch him on the ward and see if he started to deteriorate, scan him then but risk delaying treatment if he did actually have a brain bleed. The discussion seemed to go on for ever, even printing out a copy of the national guidelines for him to read, didn't seem to help.

'What would you do if it were your son?' he eventually asked.

'I would watch him and not scan,' I replied.

'Why didn't you tell me that ages ago then? We would have saved the last 20-minute discussion.'

From now on, I do.

Keeping patients up to date with what is going on

I was a patient for a couple of weeks, two years ago. There is nothing as scary and annoying as not knowing what is going. I keep this in mind with all my patients now.

Learning to communicate better with my team

I was treating a lady who worked at the local Chinese takeaway restaurant. She was having an exacerbation of her chronic respiratory condition and I made of series of requests to the junior doctor I was working with. I checked that my colleague knew what I wanted by saying 'Happy?' and her response was a nod, which I took to mean yes. On review 30 minutes later, I saw that 2 of the things requested hadn't happened – this could compromise care. I felt annoyed with her, for not listening and, I thought, not working as a team.

Then the patient said to me: 'How could you know she knew what you wanted. You didn't check with her. I have never got an order wrong in our restaurant as I always read back to the customer what I think they said. That way there is no confusion and no errors.' I paused and thought what a genius she was and what a fool I was. Now I practise the 'Chinese takeaway' style of communication whenever I am issuing or following treatment plans. I may sound like a man suffering from a compulsive disorder, but it has lead to less errors and better care.

☊ Oh shit I am pregnant

Miss S was an 18-year-old Korean girl, on holiday with her family when a sudden bout of abdominal pain had diverted her from her sightseeing fun to A&E.

She presented with all the classical signs of appendicitis: pain in the right lower abdomen, no appetite and inability to do anything that increased the pressure in her stomach, e.g. coughing etc. She also had a negative Croydon triad. (The Croydon triad is the rule that if three of the following are present, then the chances of right lower-sided pain being due to a sexually transmitted disease leading to pelvic inflammatory disease are greater than the chances of appendicitis: large hooped earrings, toe ring, ankle bracelet and small dolphin tattoo on the side of their belly/backside.)

Luckily this girl had none of these signs and I was pretty confident in my diagnosis of appendicitis. I assessed her and took blood and asked for a urine sample. It is routine procedure for any woman between 13 and 60 to have a pregnancy test if they come in with abdominal pain.

The results came back as positive. This threw my appendicitis diagnosis into question and threw up a new possibility of the pain being caused by an ectopic pregnancy. I needed to tell her the result as it meant more investigations and some of these might require an intimate examination. We hadn't actually told her that we would be doing a pregnancy test as part of the routine assessment so there was no lead in to telling her the result. I asked to have a word with her alone, without her parents, at which she looked very frightened and I realised how young for her age she seemed. I asked her gently if she thought she might be pregnant but I was met with a flat denial and an explanation that she had never even had sex as she was unmarried. She was very adamant about this. I wanted to believe her but the fact was that the test had come back positive. Falsely positive tests can happen but are very rare. I believed the test more than I believed her. Tests generally don't lie but frequently teenagers do. I told her about the results of the test. Naturally she was very shocked and upset and worried about her parents. She still denied having had sex.

Suddenly she came up with a possible explanation.

A few weeks ago her boyfriend had touched her 'down below'. She had liked the feelings but asked him to stop it as she wanted to wait till she was married. But she told me this is how she must have got pregnant. He had never actually penetrated her with anything other than his finger and that his fingers had been nowhere near his manhood before then. So I thought this was unlikely. She also asked if she could have got pregnant by giving her boyfriend a blow job, which is as far as she goes with him. I explained no and was a bit short with her. Why was she lying to me? I'd already told her I wouldn't tell her parents but she still stuck to her story that she had never had sex.

She was in tears, scared witless, I imagine. I left her for a time to have a think while I arranged her admission. I was hoping the truth would be remembered soon, otherwise I had been talking to the twenty-first-century Virgin Mary. I went to write my notes when one of the doctors was joking to one of the nurses that she had done a pregnancy test on the lady in the opposite cubicle even though she had had a hysterectomy (removal of the uterus.) two months previously.

'But it had come back positive' she exclaimed.

'Blooming heck!' I thought. What an amazing time the obstetricians are going to have for the next few months; A Virgin birth – the first one in over 2,000 years – and a pregnant woman without a uterus… What the…? Bloody hell, I thought, as it clicked into place.

I got the packet of pregnancy sticks and picked up three at random.

I went to the toilet and pissed on the first one. The pink line came up. I'm pregnant.

I tried the second. I was having twins.

We urgently needed some new testing strips. We repeated the test and it was negative. Which was fantastic for her and not so good for me. I had to tell her that all the upset and worry I had put her through was all unnecessary, it was just that our bloody pregnancy tests were faulty.

I went in humble as possible and she was there with her mum. I apologised profusely.

She was so kind about it. 'I wasn't worried for one moment as I have only ever held hands with my boyfriend.'

I smiled as I organised for the surgeons to come and review her. I had two more things to do. I wrote an incident form about the pregnancy test batch and then went to the toilet. I peed on one of the new ones. I wasn't pregnant. Phew! I had no idea how I would have explained that one away to my wife.

℞ So pleased he broke his ankle

One of the patients who has made me really happy came in with an injured ankle. He was in his 50s, a builder by trade and an absolutely delightful man. He had come in after playing football with his 3-year-old grandson. He slipped on the grass and got a small break to his fibula. An easy to treat fracture, which I was delighted he got.

The reason I was so happy was that he looked very familiar. I had been part of a team that treated him about 4 months previously. He had had an out of hospital cardiac arrest caused by a heart attack, his heart had stopped for 13 minutes and in essence he had died. A member of the public saw him collapse and immediately started chest compressions. The ambulance arrived and started his heart again using a defibrillator. When he arrived in the emergency department, I was in charge of his care. We gave special drugs to keep up his blood pressure, and we used special ice packs to cool down his body temperature to protect his brain from the damage that had occurred to his body during the arrest. He went from us in A&E to the cardiac catheter lab and had a stent placed to open up the blocked vessels. A bit like a plumber unblocking your drain. He went on to have a balloon pump placed in his aorta (largest blood vessel coming from the heart) to help keep up his blood pressure. He went from there to the ICU, where he was kept alive by dialysis despite his kidneys failing. From there he went back to the cardiology unit where he had a pacemaker fitted which not only sensed if his heart missed beats, but also controlled how frequently it beat and could also shock his heart back into a normal rhythm if he were to have another cardiac arrest.

After discharge a team of rehabilitation physios worked on him to get him up to working again and playing football with his grandson. His GP provided ongoing care, reassurance and a point of contact where all the specialists he needed could feed in.

Ten years ago, he would have died. Now he can live a full life, thanks to the advances in technology and increased funding for the NHS. At no point in this scenario did we stop to question if he had insurance or if he could pay for the treatment he received. We did not care if he was a millionaire or on the dole. All we wanted was to give him the best possible chance to walk out of the hospital, not only alive but in good enough shape to live a normal life again. This is possible because of the way the NHS works – it is free to whoever needs it regardless of ability to pay and with cooperation and not competition between the many different health care professionals and services. Thanks to the NHS he lives to fight another day. It was great to be a small cog in his care 4 months ago. It is great he has been well enough to go out and break his ankle.

The future of the NHS

I firmly believe that the last patient is alive todaybecause of the health service we have in the UK. In the USA, he wouldn't have been able to afford the costs of this expensive state of the art treatment. The ambulance service, GPs, A&E, cardiologists and intensive care team all worked together thinking about how best to care for the patient without considering how we could make a profit out of our patient. He got excellent but also efficient care because there was no incentive to do unnecessary tests to create extra profits. Health care isn't appropriate to be run like a business, where cutting costs and removing competition lead to more profits. Working together, improving quality and cooperating with local hospitals and GPs is the best way to run health services and we are lucky that we in the UK have the NHS which in essence does this.

Yes, it has it problems, but they are solvable by good management. Despite the extra resources, there has been money wasted, excessive micro-management and sledge hammers to crack nuts. This has led some doctors and nurses, and a large section of the press, to not appreciate what we do have.

Recently there has been an appreciation that the government needs to let clinicians take the lead on how to improve care. For instance, in A&E the government worked with A&E doctors and nurses about implementing new standards of quality of care and not just a time standard – the old 4-hour rule. The debacle of modernising medical careers, where good doctors were left without jobs, has largely been resolved as have reforms about improving accountability of doctors and learning from mistakes.

The ethos of the NHS – cooperation and not competition and putting patients before profits – has served us well, despite years of underfunding which has only partially been rectified in the last decade. The new reforms to the NHS in England (the NHS in Wales and Scotland are not following these reforms) are essentially following Blair's reforms but at breakneck speed, and I believe are very risky.

Although I agree that GPs should be central to commissioning health care for their patients, it is the future of hospitals that concerns me. GPs will be able to buy services from any provider; hospitals will be able compete against each other on price and as standalone institutions. The ethos of cooperation will be eroded and the NHS could just become a kite mark for an umbrella of organisations which are providing health care independently, often with the aim to make as much money as possible, rather than working together for the health of the local area.

It doesn't really matter if your local hospital stopped doing elective hip operations as the private treatment sector undercut them, but what happens at 2 a.m. when your nan has broken her leg and there is no orthopaedic doctor available in an emergency as they no longer work for the NHS? Or worse still, they are available but so inexperienced at what should be the bread and butter of their job that poor care is given in the end?

I don't honestly believe that the government wants to dismantle the NHS. I do, however, have concerns that a blind acceptance of market forces in health care could lead to the unintended consequence of a dismantling of the ethos and structures of the NHS. It is these that have served us well, from cradle to grave, regardless of ability to pay.

℞ So to round up...

This book has no firm end. The last story and the one I have chosen to end the book on wasn't special, wasn't particularly fascinating and wasn't a particularly exciting case for me – a simple fractured ankle. But for the patient it was. For him it was special; he was so anxious about his injury, the effects it would have on his job and livelihood, worried about if he would survive an anaesthetic and worried that he might never run again.

I knew he was going to be okay, but he didn't, he was scared. The words I spoke did matter and were unique for him. And he reacted differently to how other patients did and so his similar condition became a unique encounter.

I have learned a lot in the last few years. Not facts or new drugs – they can be looked up on 'Google' anyhow – but the importance of how we speak to our colleagues and our patients, how we implement what is already known about best patient care so that all our patients can get top notch treatment, and most importantly how we look after ourselves.

Medicine is an art as well as a science. Only by thinking about what we do, can we appreciate that art. This book in essence has been one long reflective practice essay. What I used to mock that medical schools taught as an unnecessary piece of political correctness, I have come to use, to help me enjoy my job and care as best I can for my patients. I go on looking forward to another 30 years of this.

Glossary

ASBO – antisocial behavioural order. I believe over 90 per cent of people coming to A&E after midnight on a Saturday night have or should have one of these.

Blair, Tony – icon of revolutionary socialist ideology or Thatcher's love-child who acts as a tree for George Bush's poodle. You choose.

BMA – British Medical Association (the doctors union) but not the type that calls each other comrade and organises meat raffles. A GP's best friend.

BMJ – *British Medical Journal* (the *Sun* of medical journals). You can understand most of the words, it keeps you vaguely interested and there is often an interesting picture or two.

Brown, Gordon – icon of revolutionary Scottish socialism or a boring and impolite version of Tony Blair. I am not sure which one yet.

Cannula – a plastic tube that goes in the back of your hand and from which we can take blood tests and give you fluids and drugs. Not really something to make a joke out of, as it has no amusing properties.

Charge nurse – nurse in charge. It is what we call male sisters. They object to the term 'brother'.

Chav – English equivalent of trailer trash. Spend money on crap food, fags and on Burberry gear.

Choose and book – to make the NHS look good we now let

you choose if you want to go to your local hospital or one 50 miles away.

Copper – policeman; precious metal.

CPR – cardiopulmonary resuscitation.

Cross matching – finding out what batch of donated blood is compatible with the patient's.

Dowie, Iain – footballer (very, very good in his time) and manager (not so good). Like all the best sportsmen he has got a big, ugly bent nose.

DGH – district general hospital. Your local hospital. Apparently our affection for them is the problem for the NHS and they must be destroyed. Personally, I think they do a good job for the populations they serve.

Diagnostic and treatment centres – New Labour term for hospitals. So we close down NHS DGHs and open these 'for profit' diagnostic and treatment centres instead. Makes sense to me. Same as independent treatment centres/private treatment centres.

DVT – deep vein thrombosis.

ECHO – echocardiogram. Takes an ultrasound picture of your heart. It looks like a fuzzy black and white TV screen. I have no idea how people can actually interpret these things.

Fast bleeped – called quickly. Response is often variable.

Frusemide – a drug that makes you pass urine. The Americans keep trying to get us to change the way we spell it, but I won't succumb to the pressure.

Fracture – exactly the same as a break.

Glomerulonephritis and **cANCA** – something to do with the kidneys but the subject went way over my head at medical school. Only properly understood by renal specialists and perhaps Einstein.

GMC – General Medical Council. They make sure that doctors are being good boys and girls and investigate when the public/colleagues complain. There is no truth whatsoever to the rumours that they have trained CIA agents working for them as undercover investigators.

GP (general practitioner) – your family doctor. They tend to come in two types: partners (good businessmen, who happen to be doctors) and salaried GPs who work for the former but don't have a financial interest in the practice (they don't own as expensive a car or do as much paper work).

GTN – a drug to help with angina.

Haemoglobin – the oxygen-carrying part of your red blood cells/ blood. Not enough and you become anaemic.

Hewitt, Patricia (Secretary of State for Health) – the doctor's and nurse's best friend. Bastion of keeping the NHS public. A great moral thinker of our time. Highly respected among all that work in the NHS. I would personally walk for miles barefoot over broken glass, just to hear her wise words…

Hoodie – a naughty boy or girl who is worried about the rain damaging their new hair-do.

ICU – intensive care unit. Also known as ITU – intensive treatment unit. The area of the hospital where the sickest patients receive specialised and life saving treatment. Nicknamed 'expensive scare unit'.

Lancet – another medical journal that gets itself into hot water a bit. Fewer pictures than the *BMJ* and longer words. Hence, has a slightly higher brow readership (*P.S The MMR jab is a good thing*).

MAU – medical admissions unit.

NHS – National Health Service. The greatest achievement of a socialist Labour government. Set up in the late 1940s to provide free care to all who need it from the cradle to the grave. Was once the envy of the world.

Naloxone – drug that reverses the effects of heroin. Helps drug users to breathe; also gets them off their high rather abruptly.

PCT – primary care trust. Holds the purse strings and power in the NHS.

PFI – private finance initiative. Another name for a very, very expensive loan that doesn't appear on the Chancellor's ledger.

Reconfiguration – New Labour speak for closing departments, wards and hospitals.

Red phone – the ambulance service use it to tell us about emergencies. Called the red phone no matter what colour it actually is.

Resus – resuscitation department. Where we take the sickest patients and where we don't get bothered about 4-hour rules (usually).

Revalidation – the GMC word for the idea to retest doctors' skills and knowledge every so often to make sure we are not like Harold Shipman.

Socialist principles – something that New Labour has very little experience of. As opposed to PFI and for-profit independent treatment centres, which it knows all about.

SHO – Senior House Officer, old term for a junior doctor in training. Now replaced by foundation doctors, specialty training doctors or unemployment.

SMINT – senior minor injury nurse triage.

Staph./Staph. aureus – a bacterium of some strength and power. Known for MRSA (methicillin resistant *Staphylococcus aureus*) and the new deadly killer MSSA (methicillin sensitive *Staph. aureus*) – otherwise known as bog standard *Staph. aureus*.